NATURAL RECIPES

Inspired by
Barbara O'Neill's Teachings

Wholesome Plant-Based Yummy Food

PrimeInsight Press

TABLE OF CONTENTS

Introduction

Welcome to Natural Recipes Inspired by Barbara O'Neill's Teachings.

Step into a world of culinary delight guided by the profound wisdom of naturopath Barbara O'Neill. This cookbook is your gateway to a multitude of wholesome recipes meticulously designed to adhere to her principles of healthy living.

Within these pages, you'll discover a diverse array of recipes tailored to suit every moment of your day. Each dish has been crafted to not only tantalize your taste buds but also align with Barbara O'Neill's profound insights into the art of healthy living. This cookbook will empower you to make mindful and nutritious choices, ensuring that your well-being is always a priority.

Barbara O'Neill's Wellness Philosophy.

Barbara O'Neill is renowned for her passion for nature and her nursing background. Her personal journey into natural healing, spurred by a significant challenge with her first child, led her to explore natural treatments and successfully experiment with them on herself and her family. Barbara believes in the body's innate self-healing and design. Her mission is to share the conditions and knowledge necessary to activate and support the self-healing power of our remarkable bodies.

Dive into a World of Nourishing Recipes.

This cookbook is more than just a collection of recipes; it's a reflection of the harmony between healthy living and delectable cuisine. You'll find an abundance of recipes covering all your daily occasions. Whether it's a hearty breakfast to start your day, a quick and nutritious lunch, or an indulgent yet health-conscious dinner, we have you covered.

Not only are these recipes delicious and easy to prepare, but they also reflect Barbara O'Neill's principles, ensuring that your culinary journey aligns with your path to a healthier and more vibrant life.

Join us in celebrating the art of self-healing through the pleasure of wholesome cooking. Dive into these recipes and let your journey toward well-being begin.

For general well-being

These are some valuable recommendations inspired by Barbara O'Neill. It's not obligatory to strictly adhere to these guidelines, but gradually integrating some of them into your daily routine can contribute to enhancing your overall health.

1. Aim to maintain proper hydration by consuming 2 to 3 liters of water daily. Be sure to enrich every cup of water with the touch of Celtic salt, a little secret to enhance the benefits of hydration.

2. Start your day with an early awakening, a small gesture that allows you to fully embrace the opportunities of the new day.

3. Kickstart your morning with a splash of vitality: a glass of fresh water infused with the scent of lemon, a refreshing touch to start the day on the right foot.

4. Make room for exercise in your daily routine, a precious investment to preserve and boost your health.

5. Gift your body with the benefit of probiotics by incorporating them into your diet through the intake of water enriched with these valuable health allies.

6. Maintain your salt balance and reap the health benefits by ensuring that Celtic salt is part of your daily water intake.

7. Dedicate a 30-minute break after morning water consumption, a moment to let your body slowly absorb this valuable resource.

8. When it's time for breakfast, don't forget to take care of your oral hygiene and experiment with coconut oil pulling, a healthy custom to start the day.

9. After breakfast, allow yourself a break of about 1.5 hours before having another sip of water. Each glass should contain the magical touch of Celtic salt, and you can sip it up to half a cup at a time.

10. Approaching lunch, remember to stop water intake about 30 minutes before sitting down to your meal.

11. About 5 hours after the first meal of the day, it's time for lunch, an opportunity to nourish your body in a healthy and balanced way.

12. After lunch, dedicate another 1.5 hours to your body's well-being before indulging in another sip of water.

13. Add a touch of variety to your day with a cup of dandelion tea or similar beverages, a delightful habit to incorporate into your routine.

14. Continue to include Celtic salt in your daily water intake, a small ritual that could have significant benefits for your body.

15. For dinner, enjoy a light portion whenever it suits your schedule. The key is to maintain a healthy balance in evening meals.

16. Ensure you get a restorative sleep by going to bed between 9 and 10 PM, a crucial contribution to your overall health.

These guidelines provide valuable support for your general well-being. While it's not necessary to follow them rigorously, gradually integrating some of these practices into your daily life can significantly enhance your health.

Eating Habits for Optimal Well-Being

Focus on the Following (80% of Your Diet):

- Prioritize alkaline foods.

- Choose organic options when possible.

Incorporate These Foods Regularly:

- Lemon

- An abundance of dark green vegetables

- Lima beans

- Lentils

- Unrefined coconut and extra virgin olive oils

- A variety of fruits

- Nutrient-rich grains such as millet, quinoa, amaranth, sorghum, spelt, and kamut

- Almonds and Brazilian nuts

- A diverse selection of seeds including chia, pumpkin, hemp, and sunflower

- Include soy-based products like milk and tofu

Occasional Indulgences (20% of Your Diet):

- Consume these foods less frequently to maintain a balanced diet.

Enjoy in Moderation:

- Other cereals not mentioned earlier

- Additional legumes not previously listed

- Nuts not covered in the previous category

- Rice, preferably basmati

- Eggs

- Goat milk

- Fresh cheese options such as fetta and ricotta

- Fermented products like miso, kefir, yogurt, kombucha

- Natural sweeteners such as honey, maple syrup, coconut/palm sugar, rice malt, and stevia

- Mushrooms

- A variety of herbs and spices

- Carob powder

- Sparkling water

- Tahini

- Sprouts

Maintaining a diet rich in alkaline foods and emphasizing organic choices when available can promote overall well-being. While the first category forms the foundation of your nutrition, the second category offers flexibility for occasional indulgences.

Aim to Minimize:

- Reduce consumption of the following items.

Choose Sparingly:

- Meat

- Seaweed

- Crayfish and lobsters

- Nutritional yeast

- Dairy, particularly cow's milk

- Cinnamon

Eliminate Completely:

Completely remove these items from your dietary intake for optimal well-being.

- Refined sugar

- Alcohol

- Drugs

- Spicy condiments like chili, mustard, black and white pepper

- Hybridized wheat

- Store-bought peanuts

- Caffeinated beverages, including green tea, matcha, and cacao

- Tobacco

- Table salt

- All types of vinegar

- Fermented foods

- Aged cheeses

- Vegetable oils, including canola

Conscious food choices can contribute to your overall sense of well-being. By minimizing certain items and eliminating others, you can support a healthier lifestyle.

BREAKFAST

Nutty Breakfast Bars

Ingredients:

- 260g shredded coconut

- 1/2 cup of pumpkin (pepita) seeds

- 1/2 cup of sunflower seeds

- 1/2 cup of flaxseed (linseed)

- 6 dried figs or Medjool dates, roughly chopped

- 1 teaspoon of ground cardamom

- 4 tablespoons of tahini

- 3-4 tablespoons of maple syrup or raw honey

- 4 tablespoons of psyllium husks

- 2 tablespoons of filtered water

- A pinch of Celtic salt

Instructions:

1. Process the shredded coconut in a high-speed blender or food processor until it reaches a creamy, butter-like consistency.

2. Add the remaining ingredients and pulse until they are thoroughly combined.

3. Line a slice tray with greaseproof paper. Spread the mixture evenly over the tray, pressing it down to reach the edges. Place another sheet of greaseproof paper on top and use a second tray to press down on the mixture to flatten it evenly.

4. Use a sharp knife to mark the flattened mixture into 20-25 bars.

5. Keep the bars in the freezer and enjoy them for breakfast or as a snack. Serve them directly from the freezer.

Nutritional Information (per bar - makes 20-25 bars): Calories - 137, Protein: 3g, Carbohydrates: 13g, Fat: 9g

Nutty Banana Buckwheat Cereal

Ingredients:

- 1 cup of cooked buckwheat cereal

- 1/4 cup of creamy coconut milk

- 1 tablespoon of almond butter

- 2 tablespoons of chia seeds

- 2 tablespoons of sliced almonds

- 1/2 of a sliced banana

- 1/2 scoop of protein powder

- Nutrient highlights: Fiber, Protein, Healthy Fats

Instructions:

1. Combine cooked buckwheat cereal, creamy coconut milk, almond butter, chia seeds, and sliced almonds in a bowl.

2. Top with sliced banana and a scoop of protein powder.

3. Enjoy your nutrient-rich and delicious bowl of Nutty Banana Buckwheat Cereal!

Nutritional Information (per serving): Calories - 325, Protein: 11g, Carbohydrates: 34g, Fat: 17g

Homemade Gluten-Free Buckwheat Granola

Ingredients:

Dry Mix:

- 3 cups of coconut flakes

- 3 cups of almond flakes

- 1 cup of chia seeds

- 2 cups of soaked and drained buckwheat

- Nuts and seeds of your choice.

Wet Mix (Granola)

Ingredients:

- 150ml of coconut cream

- 1 tsp of vanilla extract

- 1 tsp of your preferred spices (such as cardamom, ginger, or Ceylon cinnamon)

- Optionally, you can add maple syrup, orange juice, or lemon zest

Instructions:

1. Soak the buckwheat for 3 hours, then rinse and drain it.

2. In one bowl, combine all the dry ingredients. In a separate bowl, mix the wet ingredients. Coat the dry mixture with the wet ingredients, ensuring it's well-coated without being overly soaked. Add more liquid as needed.

3. Bake the mixture at 180°C (350°F) for 25-30 minutes, checking and stirring every 10 minutes to prevent burning.

4. Alternatively, you can place it in a dehydrator overnight.

5. Once it's cooled, you can add dried fruit if desired.

6. Store the granola in an airtight container. Enjoy it as a topping for fruit, yogurt, or pear cream, or simply savor it with any plant-based milk as a wholesome breakfast cereal.

Nutritional Information (per serving, assuming 6 servings): Calories - 216, Protein: 4g, Carbohydrates: 23g, Fat: 13g

Protein-Packed Apple Oatmeal

Ingredients:

- 1 cup of oatmeal

- 2 cups of water

- 1/8 tsp of pink salt

- Half a chopped apple

- 1/4 cup of coconut milk

- 1/2 scoop of sugar-free plant protein powder (providing 10 grams of protein)

- 1 tbsp of almond butter

- 1/4 cup of chopped walnuts

- 2 tbsp of chia seeds

- Drizzle of honey

Instructions:

1. In a slow cooker, combine oatmeal, water, pink salt, and half a chopped apple. Cook until the oatmeal is soft and well-cooked.

2. Stir in the coconut milk and sugar-free plant protein powder.

3. Top the oatmeal with almond butter, chopped walnuts, chia seeds, and the remaining half of the chopped apple.

4. Drizzle honey over the oatmeal. This protein-packed oatmeal provides about 27 grams of protein, making it an ideal breakfast option.

Nutritional Information (per serving, assuming 1 serving): Calories - 407, Protein: 27g, Carbohydrates: 46g, Fat: 15g

Zucchini Corn Fritters

Ingredients:

2 cups freshly grated zucchini (approximately 2 medium zucchinis)

1 cup sweet corn kernels

1/4 cup finely chopped shallots

1 1/4 cups chickpea flour

1 tsp baking powder

1 tsp smoked paprika

1/2 tsp garlic powder

1/2 tsp onion powder

1/2 cup non-dairy milk

2 flax eggs (2 tbsp flaxmeal mixed with 5 tbsp water)

1/4 tsp Celtic salt

Instructions:

Preheat the oven to 180°C (350°F) and line a baking tray. Use a clean kitchen towel to squeeze out excess moisture from the grated zucchini.

In a mixing bowl, combine all the ingredients thoroughly.

Spoon the mixture onto the baking tray, and lightly spray them with cooking spray. Bake for 35-40 minutes, turning them halfway through until they are golden brown.

Serve the zucchini corn fritters warm. They go great with your favorite dipping sauce or as a side to a fresh salad.

Serving Size - 1 fritter. Calories: 87, Fat: 2.7g, Carbohydrates: 13.8g, Fiber: 2g, Protein: 3g

Vegan Cashew Cream Cheese

Ingredients:

Yields 1 cup

1 cup raw cashews (soaked for at least 4 hours if you don't have a high-powered blender)

1/2 cup water

1.5 tbsp lemon juice

Heaping 1/4 tsp Celtic salt

If you soaked your cashews, be sure to drain and rinse them thoroughly until the water runs clear.

Instructions:

In a blender, combine all the ingredients and blend until a smooth and creamy consistency is achieved.

You can serve this cashew cream cheese immediately or chill it for later use. When chilled, it will thicken up slightly, but you can thin it with a small amount of water if needed.

Leftovers can be kept in the fridge for about 5 days.

Serving Size - 2 tablespoons. Calories: 86, Fat: 7g, Carbohydrates: 4g, Fiber: 1g, Protein: 2g

Spicy Vegan Breakfast Sausage Patties

Ingredients:

- 1 cup old-fashioned oats

- 1/4 cup ground flaxseeds

- 1/4 cup chia seeds

- 2 tbsp miso paste

- 1 tbsp onion powder

- 1 tbsp garlic powder

- 1 tbsp maple syrup

- 2 tsp paprika

- 2 tsp oregano

- 1 tsp ground sage

- 1 tsp ground fennel

- 1 tsp dried thyme

- 1 tsp cumin

- 1/2 tsp Celtic salt

- 1/4 tsp cayenne pepper

- 3/4 cup vegetable stock

- 3 tbsp tamari

- 1 tsp liquid smoke

Instructions:

1. In a mixing bowl, combine the dry ingredients and mix well.

2. Add the wet ingredients and continue mixing until well combined. The mixture should come together and hold its shape.

3. Allow the mixture to sit for 10 minutes to let the chia seeds and flaxseeds absorb moisture.

4. Preheat the oven to 180°C/350°F.

5. Place the sausage patties on a greased and lined oven tray.

6. Bake for 30 minutes, flipping them halfway through baking.

7. This recipe yields 12 patties.

Nutritional Information (per serving - 1 patty): Calories - 65, Fat: 3g, Carbohydrates: 7g, Fiber: 2g, Protein: 3g

Homemade Sourdough Bread

Ingredients:

- 1/2 cup sourdough starter

- 1/2 cup spelt flour

- 1/4 cup lukewarm water

- 3 cups all-purpose flour

- 1 1/2 cups lukewarm water

- 1 tbsp olive oil

- 1/4 tsp salt

Instructions:

1. Combine the sourdough starter, spelt flour, and 1/4 cup lukewarm water. Stir and let it sit covered for 24 hours or until it becomes "bubbly."

2. Once it has doubled or tripled in volume, place it in a stand mixer with a dough hook.

3. Add 3 cups of all-purpose flour, 1 1/2 cups lukewarm water, olive oil, and salt to the mixer.

4. Mix until the dough is well combined and comes away from the sides of the bowl.

5. Cover the dough and let it sit for about 4 hours.

6. Remove the dough from the bowl, shape it into loaves, or place it in a bread pan. Let it rise for 3 hours.

7. Preheat the oven to 425°F.

8. Bake the bread for about 25 minutes.

Nutritional Information (per 2 oz serving): Calories - 85, Fat: 1g, Carbohydrates: 17g, Fiber: 1g, Protein: 3g

Red Lentil Dahl

Ingredients:

- 2 cups red lentils, rinsed and drained

- 2 tsp Celtic salt

- 2 tsp turmeric

- 2 tsp Italian herbs

- 4 tbsp olive oil

- Fresh coriander for garnish

Instructions:

1. Bring the red lentils to a boil and rinse them again.

2. Cover the lentils with fresh water and cook on low heat for 15 minutes.

3. Add the turmeric, Italian herbs, salt, and olive oil. Mix well.

4. Serve as a savory breakfast dish on top of sourdough spelt toast with avocado. Garnish with fresh coriander.

Nutritional Information (per 4 oz serving without toast): Calories - 310, Fat: 14g, Carbohydrates: 33g, Fiber: 4g, Protein: 14g

Vanilla Chia Pudding

Ingredients:

- 1/4 cup chia seeds

- 2 tbsp maple syrup

- 1 tsp vanilla extract

- 1 cup almond milk

Instructions:

1. In a bowl, combine chia seeds, maple syrup, and vanilla extract.

2. Add almond milk to the mixture and stir thoroughly.

3. Cover the bowl and refrigerate for at least 4 hours, or overnight, to allow the chia seeds to absorb the liquid and form a pudding-like consistency.

4. Serve the vanilla chia pudding with your choice of toppings, such as fresh fruits, nuts, or a drizzle of honey, if desired.

Nutritional Information (per serving): Calories - 180, Fat: 8g, Carbohydrates: 24g, Fiber: 7g, Protein: 4g

Apple Stew

Ingredients:

- 5 Gala or another sweet apple, peeled and thickly sliced

- 2 tbsp water

- Nonstick skillet with lid

Instructions:

1. Slice the apples using an apple slicer or by hand and place them in your skillet.

2. Add the water and cook over medium-high heat. Add more water as needed to prevent burning. It's okay if they slightly caramelize.

3. Feel free to enhance the flavor by adding lemon juice, coriander, or vanilla mixed into the water.

4. Enjoy these apple slices as a delightful addition to your breakfast, paired with grains, fruit salad, or pear cream.

Nutritional Information (per serving): Calories - 90, Fat: 0g, Carbohydrates: 24g, Fiber: 4g, Protein: 0g

Tofu Scramble

Ingredients:

- 350g firm tofu

- 2 tsp grated garlic

- 2 tsp grated ginger

- 1-2 tsp Celtic salt

- 1 1/2 tsp turmeric

- 1 tsp Italian herbs

- 1/4 cup chopped parsley

- 4 tbsp water

- 2 tbsp olive oil

Instructions:

1. Start by crumbling the firm tofu and combine it with grated garlic, ginger, Celtic salt, turmeric, Italian herbs, chopped parsley, and water.

2. Cook the mixture over medium heat for about 5 minutes.

3. Just before serving, add the olive oil.

4. This flavorful tofu scramble is suitable for 6-8 servings.

Nutritional Information (per serving): Calories - 90, Fat: 6g, Carbohydrates: 5g, Protein: 6g

Delightful Homemade Granola

Ingredients:

- 9 cups rolled oats

- 1.5 cups coconut flakes

- 3/4 cup chopped pecans

- 3/4 cup slivered almonds

- 3/4 cup chopped walnuts

- 1.5 cups pineapple juice

- 1 cup extra light olive oil

- 1 cup maple syrup

- 1 tbsp vanilla extract

Instructions:

1. Start by mixing the rolled oats, coconut flakes, chopped pecans, slivered almonds, and chopped walnuts in a large bowl.

2. In a separate bowl, combine the pineapple juice, extra light olive oil, maple syrup, and vanilla extract.

3. Pour the liquid mixture over the dry ingredients and mix thoroughly with your hands.

4. Spread the mixture in 9x13 pans.

5. Bake in the oven at 170-200°F for approximately 6-8 hours.

6. Once cooled, store your granola in an airtight jar for a couple of weeks.

Nutritional Information (per serving): Calories - 260, Fat: 17g, Carbohydrates: 23g, Protein: 5g

Homemade Oven-Baked Granola

Ingredients:

- 3 cups quick oats

- 6 cups rolled oats

- 1 1/2 cups coconut chips or flakes

- 3/4 cup chopped pecans

- 3/4 cup chopped or slivered almonds

- 3/4 cup chopped walnuts

- 1 1/2 cups pineapple juice (or other fruit juice)

- 1 cup extra light olive oil

- 1 cup maple syrup

- 1 tablespoon vanilla extract

Instructions:

1. Mix the dry ingredients together, then add the liquid ingredients and mix well using your hands.

2. Spread the mixture in a 9x13-inch baking pan.

3. Bake at 170-200°F for approximately 6-8 hours until it's nicely browned.

4. Allow it to cool and store in an airtight container.

Nutritional Information (per 1/4 cup serving): Calories - 180, Fat: 11g, Carbohydrates: 17g, Protein: 3g

Delicious Coconut Yogurt

Ingredients:

- Flesh of 1 young coconut

- 1/3 cup of coconut water

- 1/2 cup raw cashews

- 1 teaspoon maple syrup

- A pinch of Celtic salt

Instructions:

1. Open the young coconut and drain the water into a bowl. Measure out 1/3 cup and reserve the rest for smoothies or other uses.

2. Scoop out the flesh from the coconut using a spoon.

3. In a blender, combine the coconut flesh, coconut water, cashews, maple syrup, and salt. Blend until the mixture is smooth.

4. This recipe yields approximately 1 1/2 cups of delicious coconut yogurt.

Nutritional Information (per serving - 1/2 cup): Calories - 226, Fat: 18g, Carbohydrates: 13g, Protein: 5g

Fruity Smoothie Bowl

Ingredients:

- 1.5 cups frozen blueberries

- 1 cup frozen raspberries

- 1 1/4 cups water or soy milk

- 1 tbsp orange juice

- 2-3 tbsp pea protein

- 1 cup ripe banana

- 2 cups baby spinach

- 1/2 cup sliced seasonal fruit

- 1 cup ripe banana, extra

- Goji berries (optional)

Instructions:

1. In a blender, combine the frozen blueberries, raspberries, 1 cup of banana, baby spinach, orange juice, pea protein, and water or soy milk (add water or milk in parts to achieve the desired thickness).

2. Purée the mixture until it's smooth.

3. Divide the smoothie into 3 bowls and top each with the extra ripe banana, seasonal fruit, and optional goji berries.

4. This recipe serves 3.

Nutritional Information (per serving): Calories - 254, Fat: 3g, Carbohydrates: 51g, Protein: 9g

Quinoa Sausage Links

Ingredients:

- 1 cup quinoa, cooked according to package instructions, washed and well-drained

- 1/2 cup oat flour

- 4 tbsp pecan meal

- 1 tbsp soy sauce

- 1 tsp garlic powder

- 1 tsp onion powder

- 1 tsp ground sage

- 1/2 tsp ground thyme

- 1/2 tsp dried rosemary

- 1/2 tsp paprika

- 1 tsp miso

- 1 tbsp water

- 1 tbsp olive oil

- 2 tsp honey

Instructions:

1. In a large bowl, combine all the ingredients thoroughly using your hands.

2. Take a heaped tablespoon of the mixture and roll it into a sausage shape approximately 7.5cm long.

3. Heat olive oil in a pan and fry the sausage links, turning them until they are evenly cooked.

4. Alternatively, you can cook them in an air fryer.

5. This recipe makes 12-16 quinoa sausage links.

Nutritional Information (per serving - 2 links): Calories - 208, Fat: 10g, Carbohydrates: 25g, Protein: 6g

LUNCH-DINNER

Savory Chickpea and Veggie Loaf

Ingredients:

- 3 tablespoons of olive oil or water for oil-free cooking

- 1 large diced onion

- 4 small diced carrots

- 3 small diced celery stalks

- 5 minced garlic cloves

- 3 cups of canned or cooked chickpeas, drained and rinsed

- 1 to 1 & 1/2 cups of breadcrumbs (use gluten-free or sourdough if desired)

- 3 tablespoons of ground flaxseeds (linseeds)

- 1 tablespoon of tamari

- 1 teaspoon of Celtic salt

- 3 tablespoons of Worcestershire sauce (use liquid smoke as an alternative)

- 1/2 cup of ketchup

Topping:

- 1/2 cup of ketchup

- 2 teaspoons of Worcestershire sauce

Instructions:

1. Preheat your oven to 180°C and lightly grease a 23cm loaf pan with olive oil or line the bottom with parchment paper to prevent sticking.

2. In a skillet, sauté the diced onion, carrots, celery, and minced garlic in olive oil or water over medium heat for approximately 5 minutes until the onions become translucent. Remove from heat and set aside.

3. In a large bowl, mash the chickpeas with a potato masher (or fork) to a slightly chunky consistency. Avoid over-mashing. Alternatively, use a food processor but pulse a few times to prevent over-blending.

4. Combine the cooked vegetables and all the other ingredients with the chickpeas. You might need an extra 1/2 cup of breadcrumbs if the mixture is too moist. Mix until well combined.

5. Press the loaf mixture into the prepared pan evenly, cover it with baking paper or foil, and bake for 30 minutes.

6. In a small bowl, mix together the ketchup and Worcestershire sauce for the topping.

7. After 30 minutes, remove the covering and spread the ketchup topping evenly on the loaf. Bake for another 15 minutes, uncovered.

8. Remove from the oven and allow it to rest for at least 15 minutes before slicing. This will help it hold together better. Optionally, sprinkle with fresh parsley before serving.

Nutritional Information (per serving - 1/4 loaf): Calories - 334, Protein: 12g, Carbohydrates: 44g, Fat: 12g

Spiced Lentil Stew

Ingredients:

- 2 tablespoons of olive oil

- 1 large onion, chopped

- 2 carrots, sliced

- 3 cloves of garlic, minced

- 1 teaspoon of grated ginger

- 2 teaspoons of curry powder

- 1 teaspoon of turmeric powder

- 1 teaspoon of ground cumin

- 1/4 teaspoon of cayenne pepper

- 6 cups of vegetable broth

- 400g can of crushed tomatoes

- 1 cup of dry green or brown lentils

- 450g of potatoes, peeled and cut into bite-size chunks

- 150g of kale or spinach, chopped

- 1 teaspoon of Celtic salt

- Lime (optional, for squeezing on top)

Instructions:

1. Heat olive oil in a large pot. Add chopped onions and sliced carrots, and sauté gently for 3 minutes.

2. Add minced garlic, grated ginger, curry powder, turmeric, cumin, and cayenne. Sauté for an additional minute, stirring often.

3. Add vegetable broth, crushed tomatoes, rinsed dry lentils, potatoes, kale or spinach, and season with salt. Cover with a lid, bring to a boil on high heat, then crack the lid slightly and simmer on medium heat for approximately 30 minutes or until the lentils are cooked. Stir occasionally.

4. Taste and adjust the seasoning with salt and spices. Serve the stew in bowls with a squeeze of lime or lemon on top and, optionally, garnish with fresh cilantro or parsley.

Nutritional Information (per serving): Calories - 268, Protein: 11g, Carbohydrates: 42g, Fat: 7g

Seasoned Tofu Taco Filling

Ingredients:

- 1 tablespoon of oil

- 1 tablespoon of soy sauce

- 1 teaspoon of smoked paprika

- 1/2 teaspoon of cumin

- 1/2 teaspoon of onion powder

- 1/2 teaspoon of garlic powder

- 1/4 teaspoon of cayenne

- 3/4 to 1 1/4 cups of salsa

- 350g of extra firm organic tofu

Instructions:

1. Preheat the oven to 180°C / 350°F. Line a large baking sheet with parchment paper.

2. Combine oil, soy sauce, and all the spices in a large bowl, creating a paste-like mixture.

3. Crumble the extra firm tofu into the bowl with the seasoning. Ensure that the tofu crumbles are evenly coated with the seasoning. Spread them evenly on the baking sheet.

4. Bake for 30 to 35 minutes, stirring the tofu occasionally. Keep a close eye on it towards the end to prevent burning. The smaller crumbles will be darker, providing a variety of textures

5. Remove the tofu from the oven and mix it with 3/4 cup of salsa. Adjust the amount of salsa to your preference, depending on the salsa's thickness and how moist you want the tofu crumbles. Heat through and serve with your choice of toppings.

Note: You can store this vegan tofu taco filling in an airtight container in the fridge for 3-4 days. It can be used in recipes that call for minced meat.

Nutritional Information (per serving): Calories - 130, Protein: 12g, Carbohydrates: 4g, Fat: 8g

Spelt Sourdough Focaccia

Ingredients:

- 50–75g of active and bubbly sourdough starter

- 375g of warm water

- 20g of honey

- 500g of spelt flour

- 9g of fine sea salt

- 2–3 tablespoons of olive oil for coating the pan

- Assorted Toppings (optional): rosemary, garlic cloves, flaky Celtic salt, tomatoes, olives, etc.

Instructions:

1. Decide when you want to prepare the dough; you can opt for a long, overnight rise at around 20-21°C / 68-70°F, or a daytime rise. Refer to the suggested schedules in the post and choose the one that suits your schedule.

2. In the evening, whisk together the sourdough starter, warm water, and honey in a large bowl. Add the spelt flour and salt. Mix until combined, and then knead by hand to form a rough, wet, and sticky dough. Cover and let it rest for 30 minutes to an hour.

3. Return to the dough and shape it into a ball.

4. For the bulk rise, cover the dough with lightly oiled plastic wrap or transfer it to an oiled dough container. Let it rise overnight at room temperature (around 20-21°C / 68-70°F) for approximately 12+ hours, or until the dough doubles in size (or more).

5. In the morning, pour 2 tablespoons of olive oil onto a rimmed sheet pan (or 1 tablespoon if using a non-stick rectangular pan). Coat the bottom and sides evenly with your hands. Place the dough on the pan, and flip it to coat both sides with your oiled hands. Cover and let it rest for 1 1/2 to 2 hours until it becomes very puffy. Preheat your oven to 220°C / 450°F.

6. Just before baking, gently press dimples into the dough using oiled fingertips, starting at the bottom and working your way to the top. As you dimple, the dough will naturally stretch outwards, forming a rustic rectangular or oval shape (about 14 x 9 inches or larger). The dough doesn't need to reach the corners and sides of the sheet pan; this is fine. You can press optional toppings; for instance, if using olives, press them into half of the pan. Sprinkle oregano evenly over the entire focaccia.

Nutritional Information (per serving - 1/8 of the focaccia): Calories - 185, Protein: 4g, Carbohydrates: 35g, Fat: 3g

Homemade Baked Beans

Ingredients:

- 2 cups of navy beans (soaked overnight)

- 2 cups of vegetable broth

- 1 cup of water

- 2 teaspoons of Worcestershire sauce

- 6 tablespoons of ketchup

- 2 tablespoons of tomato paste

- 3 tablespoons of coconut sugar

- 1 tablespoon of lemon juice

- 1 teaspoon of garlic powder

- 1 teaspoon of onion powder

- 1 teaspoon of Celtic salt

Sauce Thickening:

- 8 teaspoons of cornflour

- 1/4 cup of water

Instructions:

1. Cook Beans: Soak the navy beans in a large bowl of water for 8 to 24 hours, rinsing them multiple times. Place the beans in a large pot of water over high heat, bring to a simmer, and skim off any foam.

Reduce heat to a gentle simmer. Partially cover with a lid and cook for 1 to 1.5 hours until the beans are just tender, with a slight firmness inside (they will cook more in the sauce). Drain and rinse them again.

2. Baked Beans: In a pot, combine all the Baked Beans ingredients (except beans) and stir. Add the cooked beans.

3. Bring the mixture to a simmer, then lower the heat to medium-low and simmer for 20 minutes without a lid. Stir occasionally to prevent the beans from sticking to the pot.

4. Thickening Sauce: Mix the cornflour with water, pour it into the pot while stirring, and cook for 2 minutes until the sauce thickens (it will thicken quickly).

5. Storage: Store in the fridge for up to 5 days or freeze for up to 3 months. If the sauce becomes too thin after freezing, reheat it with a cornflour/water slurry. Typically, sauces thickened with cornflour, as opposed to flour, may lose some thickening power after freezing.

Nutritional Information (per serving - 1/2 cup): Calories - 174, Protein: 6g, Carbohydrates: 37g, Fat: 1g

Korean-Inspired Mung Bean Fritters

Ingredients:

- 2 cups of soaked and peeled mung beans

- 1 cup of water

- 1 tablespoon of toasted sesame seeds

- 1 teaspoon of garlic powder

- 1 teaspoon of onion powder

- 1 teaspoon of Celtic salt

- 1 teaspoon of miso paste

- 10 snow peas

- 3 spring onions

- 1/2 of a green bell pepper

- 1 carrot

- 1/2 of a red bell pepper

- 1/2 of an onion

Instructions:

1. In a blender, combine the mung beans, water, sesame seeds, salt, miso paste, garlic and onion powder. Blend until you have a smooth mixture.

2. Shred or slice the vegetables.

3. In a large bowl, combine all the ingredients, including the blended bean mixture and the shredded vegetables. Mix thoroughly.

4. Drop spoonfuls of the mixture into a greased frying pan and cook over low heat until they become golden brown on both sides.

Note: To prepare the mung beans, soak 1.5 cups of mung beans in 3 cups of water for about 6 hours. Remove the bean skins by rubbing the beans between your hands in a bowl of water. As the skins rise to the top, pour them off. Repeat the process until all the skins are removed.

Nutritional Information (per 3 fritters): Calories - 245, Protein: 10g, Carbohydrates: 42g, Fat: 3g

Jacquie's Baked Mung Bean Patties

Ingredients:

- 1 cup of mung beans, soaked overnight

- 1/2 cup of brown basmati rice, soaked overnight

- 1/2 cup each of grated carrot and zucchini

- 1/4 cup of chopped spring onions

- 1/2 cup of shredded red cabbage

- 1 teaspoon of cayenne pepper

- 1/4 cup of olive oil

- 1/4 cup of lemon juice

- 1/4 cup of water

- 1 teaspoon of grated fresh ginger

- 1 teaspoon of cumin powder

- Celtic salt to taste

Instructions:

1. Mix the lemon and water with the shredded vegetables and let them stand for 2-3 hours. Reserve 1/2 cup of the liquid. Set both the vegetables and the reserved liquid aside.

2. Place the soaked mung beans, rice, the reserved vegetable juice, salt, and cayenne pepper in a food processor. Process until you achieve a creamy white texture. Transfer this mixture to a bowl.

3. Add the reserved vegetables to the mixture and mix well into the batter.

4. Preheat the oven to 200°C / 350°F, shape the mixture into patties, and place them on a lined tray. Brush them with oil and bake for 35 minutes, turning them halfway through the baking process.

Nutritional Information (per patty - makes about 6 patties): Calories - 190, Protein: 4g, Carbohydrates: 28g, Fat: 7g

Homemade Legume-Based Tofu

Ingredients:

- 3/4 cup of dried beans

- Sufficient boiling water to cover the beans

- 2 and 3/4 cups of water

- 1 teaspoon of Celtic salt

Instructions:

1. Place the dried beans in a sieve and rinse them under cold water.

2. Transfer the drained beans to a medium-sized bowl and add enough boiling water to cover the beans by approximately 1/2 inch (about 1.25 cm). Allow them to sit for 20 minutes until the beans slightly swell and the water cools.

3. Drain and rinse the beans in a sieve, discarding the soaking water.

4. Place the drained beans, 2 and 3/4 cups of tap water, and optional salt in a blender. Blend on high speed until the mixture is entirely smooth, pausing to scrape down the sides of the blender container as needed.

5. Pour the bean mixture into a medium-size, heavy-bottomed saucepan.

6. Whisk it over medium-high heat for 6 to 8 minutes until the mixture becomes VERY THICK, glossy, and begins to pull away from the sides of the pan as you whisk (adjust the heat to medium as needed).

7. Transfer the batter into an 8-inch (20 cm) square glass or ceramic baking dish, smoothing the top (no need to oil the dish).

8. Refrigerate the tofu, uncovered, for at least 8 hours, or overnight. Alternatively, you can leave the tofu in the refrigerator for up to 5 days until you're ready to use it. Note: If your tofu hasn't set as pictured above, it means it wasn't cooked long enough. DO NOT CONSUME IT IF IT HASN'T SET.

9. Run a silicone spatula or a dull knife around the edge of the dish, then invert the tofu onto a cutting board. Cut the tofu into the desired shapes and sizes you prefer for recipes and storage in the refrigerator.

Notes & Tips:

1. Straining the Bean Mixture: It's crucial to achieve a 100% smooth mixture for proper cooking. Larger pieces won't cook properly using this method and may pose health risks. If you can't achieve complete smoothness, avoid using the mixture. Alternatively, if there are only a few small pieces, strain the mixture through a fine mesh sieve and discard the pieces.

2. High Altitude: This recipe is unlikely to work at higher altitudes. Instead of a quick soak, beans at high altitudes should be soaked for an extended time in cool water (12 to 24 hours) to ensure proper water absorption.

3. Storage: You can prepare the tofu up to 5 days ahead. Leave it in the original dish, or unmold it, cut into pieces, and store it in an airtight container in the refrigerator until you're ready to use it. Note that the tofu will become firmer the longer it sets.

4. Freezing the Tofu: Cut the tofu into cubes and place them in an airtight container. When defrosting, place the tofu in the refrigerator. The tofu will feel wet and springy when defrosted. Place the cubes between layers of paper towels to remove excess water (press gently if needed, but avoid pressing too hard, or the tofu will fall apart).

5. Extra-Firm Tofu Option: The original recipe yields firm tofu. For extra-firm tofu (ideal for frying, baking, and stir-frying), follow the recipe as directed but use only 2 and 1/2 cups of tap water in step 4.

6. Silken Tofu Option: For silken tofu, follow the recipe as directed but add 3 cups plus a tablespoon (about 680 mL) of water (instead of 2 and 3/4 cups) in step 4.

7. Tip: Use the bean-based tofu just like you would soy-based tofu in any recipe. For a neutral flavor, use white beans such as baby lima beans, Navy beans, cannellini, or Great Northern beans.

Nutritional Information (per 100g serving): Calories - 110, Protein: 7g, Carbohydrates: 20g, Fat: 0.5g

Vibrant Brown Rice Salad

Ingredients:

- 2 cups of cooked brown rice

- 6 spring onions, finely chopped

- 1 red bell pepper, finely diced

- 1 green bell pepper, finely diced

- 1 can (400g) of organic corn kernels

- 1/4 cup of currants

- 2 tablespoons of toasted sunflower seeds

- 1/4 cup of toasted and chopped cashews

Dressing:

- 1/4 cup of olive oil

- 3 tablespoons of soy sauce

- 3 tablespoons of lemon juice

- 1/2 teaspoon of Celtic salt

- 1 minced garlic clove

Instructions:

1. Combine all the ingredients for the rice salad in a large bowl.

2. Place the ingredients for the dressing in a jar, shake thoroughly, and pour it over the rice. Mix well. Serve.

Nutritional Information (per serving, assuming 6 servings): Calories - 390, Protein: 6g, Carbohydrates: 55g, Fat: 17g

Gluten-Free Brown Rice Mac and Cheese

Yield: 4-6 servings

Ingredients:

- 1 (320 g) sweet potato, peeled

- 1/2 small onion

- 1/2 cup of cashews

- 3 cloves of garlic

- 2 cups of water

- 2 tablespoons of soy sauce

- 1 tablespoon of miso

- 1 teaspoon of paprika

- 1/2 teaspoon of thyme

- 1/2 teaspoon of basil

- 1 teaspoon of Celtic salt

- 300g of gluten-free brown rice pasta

Instructions:

1. Chop the sweet potato into 3 large pieces and place them in a pot. Cover with water, bring to a boil, and cook for about 15 minutes. In the meantime, cook your pasta following the package instructions.

2. In a blender, combine all the sauce ingredients, including the cooked sweet potato. Blend for several minutes until creamy.

3. Drain the pasta, place it in a casserole dish, and pour the sweet potato sauce on top. Stir well.

4. Optional: You can bake the sweet potato mac and cheese at 400°F (200°C) for 8 minutes to thicken it further.

Nutritional Information (per serving, assuming 6 servings): Calories - 270, Protein: 6g, Carbohydrates: 47g, Fat: 6g

Indonesian Almond Sauce for Gado Gado

Ingredients:

- 6 cloves of garlic, thinly sliced

- 2 tablespoons of coconut oil

- 1 cup of ground almonds, lightly toasted

- 3 cups of water

- 3 tablespoons of tamari

- 2 tablespoons of maple syrup

- Juice of 1 lemon

- 4 slices of ginger

- 4 kaffir lime leaves

- 1 teaspoon of Celtic salt

- 1/4 to 1/2 cup of tahini (adjust to preferred thickness)

Instructions:

1. In a frying pan, sauté thinly sliced garlic in coconut oil.

2. Add lightly toasted ground almonds and stir over low heat until the aroma of toasted almonds fills the air.

3. Pour in 3-4 cups of water and add tamari, maple syrup, lemon juice, ginger, kaffir lime leaves, and Celtic salt.

4. Bring the mixture to a boil, then simmer for a few minutes until the sauce thickens.

5. Adjust the thickness by adding more tahini if it's too thin or water if it's too thick.

Nutritional Information (per 2 tablespoons serving): Calories - 70, Protein: 2g, Carbohydrates: 5g, Fat: 5g

Exquisite Eastern Vegetable Curry

Ingredients:

- 2 cups of diced pumpkin or squash

- 5 fresh tomatoes or 1 can of diced tomatoes

- 3/4 cup of chickpeas

- 3/4 cup of red lentils

- 1 medium onion, thinly sliced

- 1 small eggplant, cubed (2cm pieces)

- 1.5 cups of baby spinach leaves

- 1/2 cup of oil

- 1/3 cup of flaked almonds

- 1.5 teaspoons of Celtic salt.

Nutritional Information (per serving): Calories - 260, Protein: 10g, Carbohydrates: 33g, Fat: 11g

Vegan Vegetable Lasagna

Serves: 8-10

Ingredients:

- 300g of organic tofu, crumbled or sliced

- 1.5 cups of spinach

- 12 sheets of gluten-free lasagna pasta

Sauce:

- 3 medium onions, finely sliced

- 3 cups of fresh tomatoes, chopped or puréed

- 1/2 cup of olive oil

- 1 cup of celery, finely chopped

- 1 cup of carrots, finely diced

- 1 cup of zucchini, finely diced

- 4 cloves of garlic, crushed

Herb Mix:

- 3 tablespoons of tomato paste

- 1 tablespoon of dried basil

- 2 teaspoons of dried oregano

- 2.5 teaspoons of paprika

- 3 teaspoons of dried Italian herbs

- 2 teaspoons of garlic powder

- 2 teaspoons of Celtic salt

Creamy Sauce:

- 1 cup of sunflower seeds

- 1/2 teaspoon of paprika

- 1 teaspoon of garlic powder

- 1 teaspoon of onion powder

- 2 teaspoons of Celtic salt

- 2 tablespoons of cornflour

- Juice of 2 lemons

- 2 cups of water

- 1/4 cup of tahini

Instructions:

1. In a large saucepan, sauté the onion and garlic with a little water until tender. Add the vegetables and bring to a boil. Simmer for 30 minutes on low heat, then add the olive oil, herb mix, and salt. Simmer for an additional 5-10 minutes. Turn off the heat and set aside while you make the creamy sauce.

2. Preheat the oven to 190°C (375°F).

3. To prepare the creamy sauce, blend the creamy sauce ingredients in a high-powered blender until smooth.

4. For lasagna assembly, layer the following way in a medium-sized baking dish: sauce / pasta / tofu / spinach.

5. Repeat the layering: sauce / pasta / tofu / spinach.

6. Pour the creamy sauce over the lasagna, which will set as it bakes.

7. Bake for 60 minutes at 190°C (375°F) or until the top is golden brown.

8. Serve the Vegan Vegetable Lasagna with a green salad.

Nutritional Information (per serving, assuming 8 servings): Calories - 429, Protein: 15g, Carbohydrates: 29g, Fat: 28g

Velvety Roasted Cauliflower Soup

Serves: 4

Ingredients:

- 1 large cauliflower, cut into bite-sized florets

- 3 tablespoons of olive oil (divided)

- Celtic salt

- 1 medium red onion, chopped

- 2 cloves of garlic, minced

- 4 cups of vegetable broth

- 1 tablespoon of fresh lemon juice (adjust to taste)

- Scant 1/4 teaspoon of ground nutmeg

- 2 tablespoons of finely chopped fresh flat-leaf parsley, chives, and/or green onions (for garnish)

Instructions:

1. Preheat your oven to 220°C (425°F) and line a large rimmed baking sheet with parchment paper.

2. On the baking sheet, toss the cauliflower with 2 tablespoons of olive oil until it's lightly and evenly coated. Arrange the cauliflower in a single layer, sprinkle it lightly with salt, and bake until it's tender and has caramelized edges (about 25 to 35 minutes, tossing halfway).

3. While the cauliflower is roasting, in a Dutch oven or soup pot, warm the remaining 1 tablespoon of olive oil over medium heat. Add the chopped onion and 1/4 teaspoon of salt. Cook, stirring occasionally, until the onion softens (about 5 to 7 minutes).

4. Add the minced garlic and cook, stirring constantly, until it's fragrant (about 30 seconds), and then add the vegetable broth.

5. Reserve 4 roasted cauliflower florets for garnish and transfer the remaining roasted cauliflower to the pot. Increase the heat to medium-high and bring the mixture to a simmer, then reduce the heat as necessary to maintain a gentle simmer. Cook, stirring occasionally, for 20 minutes.

6. Remove the pot from heat and let it cool for a few minutes. Then, carefully transfer the hot soup to a blender, working in batches if needed.

7. Add the lemon juice and nutmeg, and blend again. Adjust the salt to taste, and add more lemon juice if you want it zingier.

8. Garnish the soup with the reserved roasted cauliflower and finely chopped fresh herbs. Enjoy!

Nutritional Information (per serving, assuming 4 servings, without garnish): Calories - 144, Protein: 5g, Carbohydrates: 17g, Fat: 7g

Velvety Roasted Cauliflower Soup

Serves: 4

Ingredients:

- 1 large cauliflower, cut into bite-sized florets

- 3 tablespoons of olive oil (divided)

- Celtic salt

- 1 medium red onion, chopped

- 2 cloves of garlic, minced

- 4 cups of vegetable broth

- 1 tablespoon of fresh lemon juice (adjust to taste)

- Scant 1/4 teaspoon of ground nutmeg

- 2 tablespoons of finely chopped fresh flat-leaf parsley, chives, and/or green onions (for garnish)

Instructions:

1. Preheat your oven to 220°C (425°F) and line a large rimmed baking sheet with parchment paper.

2. On the baking sheet, toss the cauliflower with 2 tablespoons of olive oil until it's lightly and evenly coated. Arrange the cauliflower in a single layer, sprinkle it lightly with salt, and bake until it's tender and has caramelized edges (about 25 to 35 minutes, tossing halfway).

3. While the cauliflower is roasting, in a Dutch oven or soup pot, warm the remaining 1 tablespoon of olive oil over medium heat. Add the chopped onion and 1/4 teaspoon of salt. Cook, stirring occasionally, until the onion softens (about 5 to 7 minutes).

4. Add the minced garlic and cook, stirring constantly, until it's fragrant (about 30 seconds), and then add the vegetable broth.

5. Reserve 4 roasted cauliflower florets for garnish and transfer the remaining roasted cauliflower to the pot. Increase the heat to medium-high and bring the mixture to a simmer, then reduce the heat as necessary to maintain a gentle simmer. Cook, stirring occasionally, for 20 minutes.

6. Remove the pot from heat and let it cool for a few minutes. Then, carefully transfer the hot soup to a blender, working in batches if needed.

7. Add the lemon juice and nutmeg, and blend again. Adjust the salt to taste, and add more lemon juice if you want it zingier.

8. Garnish the soup with the reserved roasted cauliflower and finely chopped fresh herbs. Enjoy!

Nutritional Information (per serving, assuming 4 servings, without garnish): Calories - 144, Protein: 5g, Carbohydrates: 17g, Fat: 7g

Cauliflower and Red Lentil Delight

Ingredients (Serves 2):

- 1/2 cup of dried red lentils, rinsed and drained

- 1 3/4 cups of cauliflower florets

- 3 teaspoons of curry powder

- 1 small onion, finely chopped

- 2 cloves of garlic, crushed

- 1 teaspoon of fresh ginger, finely grated

- 1/4 teaspoon of cayenne pepper (optional)

- 1 teaspoon of turmeric

- 1/2 cup of frozen peas

- 1/3 cup of baby spinach leaves

- 2 tablespoons of coconut yogurt

Instructions:

1. In a small saucepan, combine lentils, cauliflower, 2 teaspoons of curry powder, and approximately 3 cups of water. Cook over medium-high heat, bringing it to a boil. Then, reduce the heat to a simmer and cook for 10-12 minutes until the lentils are tender and the mixture thickens.

2. In another saucepan, heat oil over medium heat and sauté the onion until tender. Then, add the garlic, ginger, turmeric, and cayenne if using. Cook for an additional 2 minutes before transferring this mixture to the lentil-cauliflower pot.

3. Add the peas and spinach and cook for a few more minutes. Serve the dish topped with a dollop of coconut yogurt.

Nutritional Information (per serving, assuming 2 servings): Calories - 319, Protein: 14g, Carbohydrates: 58g, Fat: 3g

Cardamom-Spiced Chickpea Casserole

Ingredients (Serves 6-8):

- 1 medium onion, thinly sliced

- 2 cloves of garlic, minced

- 3 teaspoons of grated ginger

- 3 cups of cooked chickpeas

- 1 teaspoon of cardamom seeds

- 4 chopped tomatoes

- 1 tablespoon of tomato paste

- 2 teaspoons of Celtic salt

- 1/2 cup of chopped carrots

- 1/4 cup of olive oil

- 1 cup of finely chopped celery with leaves

Instructions:

1. In a large pot, sauté onions, garlic, and ginger until they turn lightly golden.

2. Add tomatoes, celery, carrots, olive oil, and cardamom seeds. Gently simmer for about 30 minutes.

3. Stir in the cooked chickpeas, salt, and tomato paste, then gently simmer for an additional 20 minutes.

4. Serve up this flavorful chickpea cardamom casserole for 6 to 8 servings. Enjoy!

Nutritional Information (per serving, assuming 6 servings): Calories - 238, Protein: 8g, Carbohydrates: 27g, Fat: 12g

Bountiful Three Bean Medley

Ingredients:

- 2 cans (each 15 ounces) of mixed beans (chickpeas, red kidney beans, cannellini beans), well-rinsed

- 2 celery stalks, diced

- 1/2 red onion, diced

- 1 cup of parsley, finely chopped

- 1 cucumber, seeds scooped out and diced

Dressing:

- 1/4 cup of lemon juice

- 2 tbsp of maple syrup

- 2 tbsp of water

- 1 tsp of dried oregano

- Celtic salt, to taste

Instructions:

1. Combine all the beans (chickpeas, red kidney beans, cannellini beans), diced celery, red onion, finely chopped parsley, and diced cucumber in a large bowl.

2. In a screw-top jar, combine all the dressing ingredients—lemon juice, maple syrup, water, dried oregano, and Celtic salt. Shake well.

3. Pour the dressing over the mixed beans and vegetables. Toss to ensure everything is well coated.

4. Store the salad covered in the fridge to allow the flavors to meld. This recipe serves 6 and makes for a delicious and nutritious side dish.

Nutritional Information (per serving, assuming 6 servings): Calories - 256, Protein: 11g, Carbohydrates: 47g, Fat: 2g

Mixed Bean Delight

Ingredients:

- 3 cans of assorted beans (e.g., kidney, cannelloni, black, butter beans, chickpeas)

- 1 cup of cooked fresh or frozen green beans

- 1/2 red onion, finely chopped

- 2 cloves of garlic, crushed

- 1/2 tsp of Celtic salt

- 3 tbsp of cold-pressed extra virgin olive oil

- Zest and juice of 1/2 a lemon

- Black or white sesame seeds for garnish (optional)

Instructions:

1. Drain and rinse all the canned beans thoroughly.

2. In a non-metallic bowl (e.g., glass), combine all the beans, including the cooked green beans.

3. Add the crushed garlic, chopped red onion, Celtic salt, lemon juice, and zest, as well as the olive oil.

4. Gently mix all the ingredients until well combined.

5. For an optional garnish, sprinkle with black or white sesame seeds.

6. Refrigerate the salad for 3-4 hours or overnight. Serve it chilled and savor the flavors.

Nutritional Information: Protein: 12-15g, Carbohydrates: 30-35g, Fat: 6-8g

Savory Lentil Patties with Cucumber Dill Dip

Ingredients:

Tzatziki Sauce:

- 1 cup of soy or coconut yogurt

- 1 tbsp of lemon juice

- 1 cucumber, peeled, seeded, and grated

- 2-3 crushed garlic cloves

- 1 tbsp of olive oil

- 1/4 cup of fresh dill, chopped

- Celtic salt to taste

Tzatziki Sauce Instructions:

1. In a bowl, combine all the ingredients and mix well.

2. Season the sauce to taste and refrigerate for 30 minutes before serving. This recipe yields about 1.5 cups of Tzatziki.

Lentil Burgers:

- 1.5 cups of cooked lentils

- 3/4 cup of spelt flour

- 1/4 cup of chopped onion

- 1 tbsp of tomato paste

- 2 cloves of crushed garlic

- 3 tbsp of soy sauce

- Flax egg (2 tbsp of flax meal with 5 tbsp of water)

- 1 tsp of cumin

- 1/2 tsp of onion powder

- 1/8 tsp of cayenne

- 1/2 tsp of garlic powder

- 2 tbsp of olive oil

Lentil Burgers Instructions:

1. Preheat your oven to 180°C. Line a baking tray with parchment paper.

2. Partially mash the lentils in a bowl, and then add all the other ingredients except for the olive oil.

3. Mix well and let the mixture sit for 10-15 minutes.

4. Form the mixture into burger patties and place them on the baking tray. Drizzle them with olive oil.

5. Bake for 30 minutes, turning them once halfway through the baking process.

6. Serve the lentil burgers in spelt sourdough buns with lettuce and Tzatziki sauce.

Nutritional Information: Protein: Approximately 10-15g (depending on the size of the patties), Carbohydrates: Approximately 30-35g, Fat: Approximately 10-12g

Pumpkin & White Bean Curry

Ingredients:

- 1kg of pumpkin, peeled and diced

- 1 tablespoon of olive oil

- 1 tablespoon of water

- 1 medium onion, chopped

- 2 cloves of garlic, crushed

- 1 teaspoon of freshly grated ginger

- 300g of cooked or raw asparagus, chopped

- 400g of white beans (butter beans can be used), cooked or canned

- 1/2 cup of coconut milk

- 50g of baby spinach leaves, chopped

- 1 tablespoon of fresh or dried basil, finely chopped

- 1 dessertspoon of Celtic salt

SPICE MIX:

- 1/2 teaspoon each of ground coriander, fennel, fenugreek seeds, cumin, turmeric powder, and caraway seeds

Instructions:

Sauté the onion over low heat in its own juices until it becomes clear. You can add a small amount of water if it sticks to the pan. Add the garlic, ginger, chopped pumpkin, olive oil, and water. Cook for 10 minutes with the lid on over low heat. When the pumpkin is almost cooked, add the white beans and the spice mix. Cook for a further 10 minutes with the lid on, adding a little water if needed. Finally, add the coconut milk, spinach, basil, and salt. Gently stir until everything is hot. Serves 4-5.

Nutritional Information: Calories per serving - 398, Fat: 12g, Carbohydrates: 62g, Fiber: 12g, Protein: 16g

Potato Leek Soup

Ingredients:

Canning Recipe (makes 7 quarts)

- 14 cups of diced potatoes

- 14 cups of chopped leeks

- Vegetable broth

- Celtic salt to taste (approximately 1 teaspoon per jar)

Instructions:

Place 2 cups of potatoes and 2 cups of leeks in each quart jar. Add salt (if desired, approximately 1 teaspoon per jar). Fill with vegetable broth, leaving 1 inch of headspace. Wipe the jar rims and put on seals and rings. Process at 11 lbs. pressure for 60 minutes. To serve, heat and add coconut cream or coconut yogurt if desired. Blend until smooth or leave it as is. Enjoy.

Nutritional Information: Calories per serving (1 quart) - 365, Fat: 1g, Carbohydrates: 84g, Fiber: 8g, Protein: 9g

Savory Nutmeat

This versatile dish can be used in various recipes to add a meaty texture. You can also slice it up for kid-friendly sandwiches. You can now find the ingredients for this online at kitchenware.com.au as it may not be available in local shops.

Ingredients:

- 2 cups of tomato purée

- 1 small onion, finely diced

- 2 cups of breadcrumbs

- 1/2 cup of boiling water

- 2 tablespoons of nut paste

- 2 teaspoons of mixed herbs

- 1 tablespoon of rice flour

- 1 teaspoon of Celtic salt

- 1 tablespoon of spelt flour

Instructions:

 Start by dissolving the nut paste in a small amount of boiling water. Then, mix all the dry ingredients together and pour in the tomato purée, boiling water, and add the onion. Combine well, then place the mixture in a sprayed baking tin for nut meats, leaving at least 5cm of space at the top. You can either steam it for 1.5 to 2 hours, covered, or bake it at 180C/350F, standing the tin upright for 40-50 minutes, depending on your oven. After baking, let it stand for 5 minutes, then remove the lids (top and bottom) and gently shake the tin to release the rolls onto a wire rack to cool. You can freeze them after baking.

Nutritional Information: Calories per serving - 200, Fat: 4g, Carbohydrates: 37g, Fiber: 5g, Protein: 6g

Nut-Free Cheese

Ingredients:

- 1 cup of yellow split peas, soaked overnight

- 1 teaspoon of garlic powder

- 1 tablespoon of onion powder

- 2 teaspoons of Celtic salt

- 2 tablespoons of lemon juice

- 2.5 cups of coconut milk

Instructions:

Place all the ingredients in a high-powered blender and blend until smooth. Transfer the mixture into a saucepan and cook over heat, stirring constantly, until it thickens. Transfer the mixture to a mold and refrigerate. This cheese is sliceable and can also be grated.

Nutritional Information: Calories per serving - 220, Fat: 9g, Carbohydrates: 29g, Fiber: 9g, Protein: 10g

Creamy Pumpkin Soup

Ingredients:

- 1 medium pumpkin (about 5 lbs.)

- 1 quart vegetable broth

- 1-2 cups almond milk (adjust to desired consistency)

- Salt and seasonings to taste (cinnamon, garlic powder, or cayenne pepper work well)

Instructions:

Start by cutting the pumpkin into chunks and roasting them at 375 degrees Fahrenheit for 45 minutes. Turn them and cook for an additional 10-15 minutes. Let the roasted pumpkin pieces cool, and then peel them. Place them in a 5-quart saucepan with 1 quart of vegetable broth and simmer for 10-15 minutes. Use an immersion blender or a conventional blender to blend the mixture until smooth. Adjust the consistency by adding 1-2 cups of almond milk. Season with salt and your choice of seasonings. Enjoy your creamy pumpkin soup.

(Nutritional Information (per serving): Calories - 120, Fat: 3g, Carbohydrates: 22g, Fiber: 6g, Protein: 3g)

Individual Lentil Loaves

Ingredients:

- 1 1/2 cups of cooked brown lentils

- 1 1/2 cups of cooked brown rice

- 1 1/2 cups of quick oats

- 1 cup of ground walnuts

- 1 tbsp of stock powder

- 5 medium mushrooms

- 1 1/2 cups of diced celery

- 1 medium onion, diced

- 1/2 cup of vegetable broth

- 2 tsp of Celtic salt

- 1 tbsp of onion powder

- 1 tbsp of garlic powder

- 1 tbsp of rubbed sage

- 1 tbsp of dried thyme

- 340g can of tomato paste

Instructions:

In a large bowl, mix the cooked brown rice and brown lentils with quick oats and ground nuts. Set this mixture aside.

In a separate pot, sauté the diced onion, mushrooms, and celery in vegetable broth until they are tender.

Add the remaining ingredients and mix well before turning off the heat.

Combine the sautéed vegetables with the lentil/rice mixture.

Add a can of tomato paste and ensure the mixture is well mixed.

Spoon this mixture into a lined muffin pan.

Cover the pan with a piece of aluminum foil and bake in a preheated oven at 180C / 350F for about 20-25 minutes.

Remove the foil and bake for an additional 10 minutes. The loaves are done when the top is browned, and the edges appear a little crispy.

Allow them to cool for 10-15 minutes. These loaves firm up with time, so making them a day ahead is recommended. You can warm them up in the oven or microwave the following day.

Nutritional Information (per loaf): Calories - 220, Fat: 8g, Carbohydrates: 31g, Fiber: 8g, Protein: 8g

No Tuna Chickpea Salad

Ingredients:

- 800g cooked chickpeas

- 1 shredded carrot

- 2 diced celery stalks

- 1/2 diced red onion

- 1/2 tsp Celtic salt

- 1 cup mayonnaise

- Fresh dill (optional)

Instructions:

 Start by mashing the rinsed cooked chickpeas in a food processor. Transfer them to a medium-sized bowl and combine with shredded carrot, finely diced celery stalks, diced onion, salt, and mayonnaise. Mix until well combined. Add fresh dill for extra flavor if desired.

Nutritional Information (per serving): Calories - 350, Fat: 23g, Carbohydrates: 35g, Fiber: 10g, Protein: 9g

German-Inspired Potato Soup

Potatoes are valuable in our diets due to their lutein content, which helps protect against macular degeneration.

Ingredients:

- 1 diced onion

- 2 garlic cloves

- 2.2 lbs of potatoes

- 2 diced carrots

- 1/8 celeriac, diced

- 1 sliced leek

- 1 bunch of parsley

- 6 cups of vegetable stock

- 1/2 tsp liquid smoke

- Celtic Salt to taste

Instructions:

1. Begin by sautéing the diced onions and garlic in a large pot.

2. Add all the remaining ingredients and cook until the potatoes are tender. You can test their doneness by inserting a knife; they should be soft with no resistance.

3. Use an immersion blender to purée half of the soup.

4. Season the soup with salt and garnish with parsley.

Nutritional Information (per serving): Calories - 290, Fat: 1g, Carbohydrates: 68g, Fiber: 11g, Protein: 9g

Lentil Hot Pot - Serve over mashed potatoes

Ingredients:

- 1 cup brown or puy lentils, soaked overnight

- 2-3 cups stock

- 2 tbsp olive oil

- 1 cup diced carrots

- 1 cup diced zucchini

- 1 cup diced onions

- 1 large tomato, diced

- 1 cup portobello mushrooms, diced

- 1/2 tsp turmeric

- 1/4 tsp cayenne (optional)

- 2 tbsp cornflour

Instructions:

1. Place lentils and stock in a large pot, bring to a boil, then lower the heat and simmer until lentils are soft, approximately 45 minutes.

2. Heat a pan with oil and add the vegetables, cooking until tender. Add the lentils with their liquid.

3. Mix the cornflour with a little water to make a slurry. Add it to the lentil mixture and cook until thickened.

4. Serve over mashed potatoes; it's a hit with kids!

Nutritional Information (per serving, including mashed potatoes): Calories - 350, Fat: 7g, Carbohydrates: 62g, Fiber: 12g, Protein: 13g

The Ultimate Pizza Crust

Ingredients:

- 1 cup spelt flour

- 1/2 tsp baking powder

- 1/2 cup natural coconut yogurt

- Extra flour for dusting

Instructions:

1. In a bowl, combine all three ingredients to form a dough ball.

2. Turn out the dough onto a floured surface and knead for about 5-8 minutes.

3. Roll the dough into a pizza shape and add your favorite toppings.

Note: This dough works well for pizza scrolls. If it's a bit too wet, add a little flour. The more you knead it, the better it comes together, becoming pliable and stretchy.

Nutritional Information (per serving - crust only): Calories - 150, Fat: 1g, Carbohydrates: 29g, Fiber: 4g, Protein: 8g

Chickpea "Chick-Con" Salad

Ingredients:

- 1 can of chickpeas (or soaked prepared dry)

- Remove the outer skins

- Mash to your preferred level of chunkiness

- Add salt, cayenne, onion powder, garlic powder, Old Bay seasoning, dill (approximately 1 tsp), and turmeric (1/4 tsp) - adjust measurements to taste

- Grated carrots, chopped celery, and green onion

- Approximately 3 tablespoons of vegan mayo

Instructions:

- Serve on your choice of bread with lettuce, tomato, avocado, onion, or...

Nutritional Information (per serving): Calories - 260, Fat: 11g, Carbohydrates: 30g, Fiber: 7g, Protein: 9g

Quick Lentil and Potato Poup

Ingredients:

- 1 diced onion

- 1 cup diced carrots

- 3.5 cups diced mushrooms

- 1 tbsp minced garlic

- 1 tsp dried oregano

- 1 bay leaf

- 1 cup red lentils

- 3 medium potatoes

- 3 cups water

- 14 oz can of tomato purée

- 3 tbsp vegetable stock powder

- 1 tsp honey

- 1 cup soy milk

- 1/2 cup chopped fresh parsley

- Celtic salt to taste

Instructions:

1. Heat up the electric pressure cooker and sauté onions and garlic until softened.

2. Add all the remaining ingredients except milk and parsley.

3. Pressure cook for 15 minutes, then release the pressure slowly.

4. Stir in the milk and parsley until well combined.

5. Serves 4-6.

Nutritional Information (per serving): Calories - 280, Fat: 4g, Carbohydrates: 50g, Fiber: 9g, Protein: 13g

Savory Stir-Fried Brown Rice

Ingredients:

- 1 cup shredded cabbage

- 1 cup finely diced onion

- 1 cup diced carrots

- 2 cloves garlic, minced

- 1/2 tsp dried basil

- 1/4 tsp paprika

- 1/4 cup diced bell pepper (capsicum)

- 4 cups cooked brown rice

- 1 cup peas

- 1 tsp Celtic salt (adjust to taste)

- 2 tbsp tamari (or soy sauce)

Instructions:

1. In a pan, sauté the vegetables using a little water until they are tender and crispy.

2. Add the tamari (or soy sauce), garlic, dried basil, and paprika. Simmer until all the water has evaporated, and the pan becomes dry.

3. Finally, add the cooked brown rice and toss it together with the vegetables.

4. This recipe serves 4-6.

Nutritional Information (per serving): Calories - 300, Fat: 2g, Carbohydrates: 62g, Fiber: 8g, Protein: 8g

Vegan Sweet Potato Patties

Ingredients:

- 1 cup cooked and mashed sweet potato

- 1 1/2 cups white beans, drained and rinsed

- 1/2 cup breadcrumbs (2 slices fresh)

- 1/4 cup finely chopped red onion

- 1 1/2 tsp garlic granules

- 1 tbsp miso paste (optional)

- 1/4 cup chopped fresh parsley

- 2 tbsp lemon juice

- Celtic salt to taste

- Olive oil for cooking

- Burger buns

- Optional Toppings: Lettuce, tomato slices, onion rings, avocado slices, and condiments of your choice

Instructions:

1. Preheat your oven to 375°F (190°C) and line a baking sheet with parchment paper.

2. In a large mixing bowl, combine mashed sweet potato, white beans, breadcrumbs, red onion, garlic granules, miso paste (if using), chopped parsley, lemon juice, and salt.

3. Mix the ingredients well until evenly incorporated.

4. Form the mixture into 4 to 6 patties, depending on your desired burger size.

5. Place the patties on the prepared baking sheet.

6. Lightly brush or drizzle the patties with olive oil to help them crisp up during baking.

7. Bake in the preheated oven for 20-25 minutes, flipping them halfway through, until they are golden brown and cooked through.

8. While the patties are baking, toast the burger buns.

9. Assemble the vegan sweet potato and white bean burgers with your favorite toppings.

10. This recipe serves 4-6.

Nutritional Information (per serving without buns or toppings): Calories - 180, Fat: 3g, Carbohydrates: 30g, Fiber: 6g, Protein: 10g

Mediterranean Chickpea Salad

Ingredients:

- 1 can (400g) chickpeas, drained and rinsed

- 1 cucumber, finely diced

- 200g cooked beetroot, finely diced

- 125g feta cheese, chopped

- 1 small red onion, finely diced

- Juice of a lemon

- 20g fresh dill, finely chopped

- Celtic salt and Cayenne pepper to taste

Instructions:

1. In a large bowl, combine chickpeas, diced cucumber, cooked beetroot, chopped feta cheese, finely diced red onion, and fresh dill.

2. Squeeze the juice of a lemon over the ingredients.

3. Season with Celtic salt and Cayenne pepper to taste.

4. Mix all the ingredients together until well combined.

5. Enjoy this Mediterranean chickpea salad!

Nutritional Information (per serving): Calories - 325, Fat: 12g, Carbohydrates: 43g, Fiber: 10g, Protein: 13g

Vegetable Curry Delight

Ingredients:

- 2 cups diced pumpkin

- 5 tomatoes or 1 can of diced tomatoes

- 3/4 cup chickpeas

- 1 medium onion, diced

- 3/4 cup red lentils or fresh green lentils

- 1 small eggplant, cubed

- 1 1/2 cups baby spinach leaves

- 1/2 cup olive oil

- 1/3 cup flaked almonds

- 1 1/2 tbsp Celtic salt

Curry Paste:

- 2 large cloves garlic, grated

- 1 tbsp fresh ginger, grated

- 1 cup fresh coriander

- 1 cup fresh mint

- 1 cup basil

- 1/4 cup water

Dry Spice Mix:

- 3 tsp turmeric

- 1/2 tsp caraway seeds

- 1 1/4 tsp coriander

- 1/4 tsp fenugreek seeds

- 1/8 tsp cayenne pepper

Instructions:

1. The day before, soak lentils and chickpeas several times, then cook until soft. Drain and set aside.

2. Preheat the oven to 200°C. Brush olive oil on the cut pumpkin and place it on a tray in the oven. Bake until it's golden brown.

3. In a large pot, sauté the diced onions on low heat until they're almost clear, then add the dry spice mix and cook for 3 minutes.

4. Add the tomatoes and eggplant and cook on low heat for 20 minutes.

5. Incorporate the cooked and drained lentils and chickpeas along with the blended curry paste, olive oil, and salt. Allow the mixture to gently simmer for approximately 10 minutes.

6. Gently fold through the baked pumpkin and spinach leaves.

7. Serve this delicious vegetable curry on brown rice cooked with turmeric (optional) and top it with slivered almonds.

Nutritional Information (per serving without rice): Calories - 420, Fat: 23g, Carbohydrates: 43g, Fiber: 16g, Protein: 16g

Moroccan Vegetable Stew

Ingredients:

- 1 can organic chickpeas

- 1 can organic lentils

- 1 can tomatoes

- Cauliflower florets

- Sweet potato, cubed

- Spinach leaves

- Carrots, sliced

- Zucchini, diced

- 1 onion, chopped

- Garlic cloves, minced

- 5-10 prunes

- 1 tsp ground coriander

- 1/2 tsp ground cumin

- 1/4 tsp ground ginger

- 1/4 tsp cinnamon

- Vegetable stock (enough to cover)

- Olive oil for frying

- Honey (to taste)

Instructions:

1. In a large pot, sauté chopped onions, garlic, and the ground spices in olive oil.

2. Add canned chickpeas, lentils, tomatoes, sweet potato, cauliflower, carrots, zucchini, and prunes.

3. Pour in enough vegetable stock to cover the vegetables.

4. Bring the stew to a boil, then reduce the heat and simmer until the sweet potato and carrots are cooked through.

5. Stir in honey to taste.

6. Add spinach leaves towards the end to wilt.

7. Adjust seasonings if needed, and enjoy your Moroccan vegetable stew.

Nutritional Information (per serving): Calories - 280, Fat: 5g, Carbohydrates: 49g, Fiber: 12g, Protein: 12g

Ginger Carrot Beet Salad

Ingredients:

- 3 carrots, grated

- 1 large beetroot, grated

- 1/2-inch piece of fresh ginger, peeled and grated

- 2 cloves garlic, minced

- Juice of 1 lemon

- 1 tbsp olive oil

- 1 tsp Celtic salt

Instructions:

1. Use a food processor or hand grater to grate the beets and carrots. Place the grated carrots and beets in a large bowl.

2. In a separate bowl, mix the grated ginger, minced garlic, lemon juice, olive oil, and Celtic salt.

3. Pour the ginger and garlic mixture over the grated vegetables and toss thoroughly. For best results, let the salad marinate for a couple of hours before serving.

Nutritional Information (per serving): Calories - 90, Fat: 4g, Carbohydrates: 13g, Protein: 2g

Quinoa and Kale Salad

Ingredients:

- 2.5 cups cooked quinoa or millet

- 1 bunch kale (about 8 oz.)

- 1 small cucumber, peeled and chopped

- 3 green onions, white parts, thinly sliced

- 1 tomato, diced

- 3 tbsp lemon juice

- 2 tbsp olive oil

- 1 garlic clove, minced

- 1/8 tsp cumin

- 1/2 tsp Celtic salt

Instructions:

1. Start by adding the quinoa or millet to 5 cups of water in a medium saucepan.

2. Bring to a rapid simmer, then cover and continue to simmer gently until the liquid is absorbed, about 15-20 minutes. If needed, add an additional 1/2 cup of water and continue to cook until absorbed.

3. Strip the kale leaves away from the stems and discard the stems. Cut the kale leaves into narrow strips, rinse well, and set aside.

4. In a large bowl, mix the cucumber, kale, green onions, and diced tomato.

5. Combine the vegetable mixture with the cooked quinoa or millet.

6. To make the dressing, combine lemon juice, olive oil, minced garlic, cumin, and Celtic salt in a jar. Shake together and pour over the quinoa, vegetables, and kale. Mix well and chill before serving.

Nutritional Information (per serving): Calories - 220, Fat: 8g, Carbohydrates: 32g, Protein: 7g

Sweet Corn Salad

Ingredients:

- 1 tbsp olive oil

- 1/2 tsp dried oregano

- 4-6 cups cooked corn

- Celtic salt, to taste

- 1.5 tsp curry powder

- 1/2 tsp dried turmeric

- 1/3 cup cashew mayonnaise

- 1/2 cup pimento-stuffed olives, sliced

- 1.5 cups red peppers, diced

- 1.5 cups green peppers, diced

- 1.5 cups red onion, diced

- 1 cup carrots, sliced

- 2 tbsp fresh coriander or cilantro, chopped

Instructions:

1. Heat olive oil in a pan and sauté the diced onion, peppers, and carrots until they soften, about 2-4 minutes.

2. Add the curry powder, dried oregano, and dried turmeric. Cook for a few more minutes.

3. Remove the pan from heat and transfer the cooked vegetables to a large mixing bowl.

4. Add the rest of the ingredients, including the cooked corn and cashew mayonnaise.

5. Mix all the ingredients well and store the salad in the fridge until you're ready to serve.

6. This salad serves 6-10.

Nutritional Information (per serving): Calories - 260, Fat: 11g, Carbohydrates: 39g, Protein: 4g

Sweet Potato and Corn Chowder

Ingredients:

- 150g can of coconut milk

- 1 cup chopped onion

- 1.5 cups chopped red pepper

- 350g - 400g tofu or 1.5 cups black beans

- 2 cups sweet potatoes, peeled and cubed

- 1 tsp Celtic salt

- 1/2 cup chopped celery

- 2 cups water

- 2 tbsp curry powder

- 1.5 cups frozen corn

- 2.5 tbsp lime juice

- 1/3 to half a cup of fresh coriander, cilantro, or Thai basil

Instructions:

1. In a large saucepan, heat 2 tablespoons of coconut milk and sauté the onion, celery, sweet potato, curry powder, and salt for 4-5 minutes.

2. Add the water and the remaining coconut milk. Bring to a boil.

3. Cover, reduce the heat, and simmer for 10 minutes.

4. Turn off the heat and use an immersion blender to purée the soup.

5. Add the red peppers, corn, tofu or beans, and turn the heat to medium-low.

6. Cover and cook for an additional 5 minutes to heat through.

7. Add lime juice, spinach, coriander, or cilantro, and stir until the spinach is wilted.

8. Serve with lime wedges. This recipe serves 4.

Nutritional Information (per serving): Calories - 340, Fat: 16g, Carbohydrates: 40g, Protein: 12g

Veggie Rainbow Bowl

Ingredients:

- 2 red onions, sliced

- 2 red peppers, sliced

- 4 diced carrots

- 3 tablespoons olive oil

- 2.5 cups butternut squash or pumpkin ribbons

- 5 cups cooked chickpeas

- 1 teaspoon ground coriander

- 4 cups chopped kale

- 1 crushed garlic clove

- 3/4 cups quinoa

- 3 cups vegetable stock

- 1 tablespoon sesame seeds

- Juice of one lemon

- Celtic salt to taste

Instructions:

1. Preheat the oven to 200°C (380°F).

2. In a large roasting tin, place the sliced onions, peppers, and diced carrots. Drizzle with 1 tablespoon of olive oil and roast for 20 minutes.

3. Add the butternut squash ribbons and cook for an additional 10 minutes.

4. In one corner of the roasting tin, add the chickpeas. Season with salt, ground coriander, and 1 tablespoon of olive oil.

5. In another corner, add the kale (massage it with 1 tablespoon of olive oil and crushed garlic) and roast for 4 minutes.

6. Put the quinoa in a pan with the hot vegetable stock. Bring to a boil and simmer for 15 minutes or until tender, allowing the liquid to be absorbed.

7. Divide the chickpeas, quinoa, and roasted vegetables among 4 bowls. Squeeze lemon juice evenly over the bowls and sprinkle with sesame seeds.

8. This recipe serves 4.

Nutritional Information (per serving): Calories - 460, Fat: 13g, Carbohydrates: 70g, Protein: 16g

Baked Eggplant Casserole

Ingredients:

- 3 large eggplants, sliced

- Spelt flour

- 1 large diced onion

- 2 cloves crushed garlic

- 1/2 cup water

- 4 peeled and diced tomatoes

- 1 tsp Celtic salt

- 1 tsp honey or maple syrup

- 2 tbsp tomato paste

- 1 tsp dried basil

- 1 tsp dried oregano

Instructions:

1. Sprinkle the eggplant slices with salt and let them stand for 30 minutes.

2. Meanwhile, sauté the diced onions and crushed garlic until soft. Add the remaining ingredients and simmer for 30 minutes.

3. After the eggplant has rested, wash and coat it with spelt flour. Shallow fry the eggplant slices.

4. Layer the eggplant and sauce, finishing with a sauce layer.

5. Bake at 180°C (350°F) for 45 minutes.

6. Optionally, sprinkle the top with chopped parsley or chopped macadamia nuts.

7. This recipe serves 4-6.

Nutritional Information (per serving): Calories - 260, Fat: 4g, Carbohydrates: 54g, Protein: 7g

Vegan Sloppy Joes

Ingredients:

- 1 diced green or red pepper

- 1 diced onion

- 3 tablespoons oil

- 2 portions of nut mince

- 1 cup coconut sugar

- Celtic salt to taste

- 2 cups tomato ketchup

- Dash of cayenne pepper

Instructions:

1. Sauté the diced peppers and onions until they are soft.

2. Add the rest of the ingredients and simmer for 15-20 minutes over medium-low heat.

3. This dish freezes well and can be served on buns with salad or coleslaw.

Nutritional Information (per serving): Calories - 320, Fat: 12g, Carbohydrates: 52g, Protein: 5g

Creamy Vegetable Pot pie Soup

Ingredients:

- 1 tbsp olive oil

- 1 small diced onion

- 1 shallot, thinly sliced

- 2 peeled and sliced carrots

- 3 sliced celery stalks

- 8 minced sage leaves

- 8 minced garlic cloves

- 2 cups soy milk

- 4 cups water

- 1 tsp miso

- 3 tbsp stock powder

- 10 thyme sprigs

- 1 bay leaf

- 3/4 cup frozen peas

- 1 tsp Celtic salt

- 1.5 cups cooked white beans

- 2 cups cauliflower florets

- 2 medium potatoes, peeled and cubed

Instructions:

1. Heat olive oil in a large pot and sauté the diced onion and sliced shallot for a few minutes until translucent.

2. Add carrots, celery, garlic, sliced sage leaves, and cook until fragrant.

3. Stir in soy milk, water, miso, stock powder, thyme sprigs, bay leaf, peas, Celtic salt, white beans, cauliflower, and potatoes.

4. Simmer for 15 minutes. Remove the bay leaf and thyme sprigs.

5. Take out 2 cups of the soup and blend until smooth, then return it to the pot along with the frozen peas.

6. This recipe serves 4-6.

Nutritional Information (per serving): Calories - 305, Fat: 4g, Carbohydrates: 57g, Protein: 15g

Lively Lemon Quinoa

Ingredients:

- 1 3/4 cups (375ml) vegetable stock

- 1 cup quinoa, rinsed well in a fine mesh sieve

- 1 TBSP olive oil

- Grated zest and juice of a lemon

- 3 spring/green onions, finely sliced

- Salt to taste

Instructions:

1. In a medium-sized pot, combine the quinoa and vegetable stock. Bring to a boil, then cover, reduce heat, and simmer for 15 minutes.

2. Remove from heat.

3. Stir in the olive oil, lemon zest, and lemon juice. Mix well.

4. Cover with a lid and let it stand for 10 minutes.

5. Fluff the quinoa with a fork, then add the finely sliced spring/green onions. Season with salt to taste.

Nutritional Information (per serving): Calories - 220, Fat: 7g, Carbohydrates: 32g, Protein: 7g

Sunflower Seed Burgers

Ingredients:

- 4 cups grated carrots or potatoes

- 1.5 cups mashed firm tofu

- 2 cups pecans or walnuts

- 1 large onion, finely chopped

- 3/4 cup spelt flour

- 3 cups water

- 2 tbsp stock powder

- 4 tbsp tomato paste

- 4 cups sunflower seeds

- 4 cloves garlic

- 1.5 cups breadcrumbs

- Celtic salt to taste

Instructions:

1. Blend sunflower seeds and pecans or walnuts until fine.

2. In a large bowl, combine all the ingredients and mix well.

3. Scoop the mixture into an oiled and lined tray and bake at 180°C (350°F).

4. After 20 minutes, turn the burgers over and continue cooking until they are golden brown.

5. Serve with tomato sauce or gravy. These burgers are excellent for freezing.

6. This recipe makes 30 servings.

Nutritional Information (per serving): Calories - 265, Fat: 17g, Carbohydrates: 19g, Protein: 9g

SNACKS-APPETIZERS

Fresh Tomato Salsa

Ingredients:
- 12 large tomatoes, halved and seeded (divided)
- 2 tablespoons of olive oil (divided)
- 1 bunch of fresh cilantro (coriander), trimmed
- 1/4 cup of lime juice
- 4 garlic cloves, peeled
- 2 teaspoons of grated lime zest
- 1 large sweet yellow pepper, finely chopped
- 12 spring onions, thinly sliced
- 1 tablespoon of ground cumin
- 1 tablespoon of smoked paprika
- 1/4 to 1/2 teaspoon of cayenne pepper
- 2 teaspoons of Celtic salt

Instructions:
1. Preheat the oven to 180°C / 350°F.

2. Place 6 tomatoes cut side down on a 15x10x1-inch baking pan and drizzle them with 1 tablespoon of oil. Roast them in the oven for 30 minutes, until the skin is blistered. Let them cool slightly.
3. In a food processor, process the uncooked and roasted tomatoes in batches until they reach a chunky consistency. Transfer all the processed tomatoes to a large bowl.
4. In the same food processor, combine cilantro (coriander), lime juice, garlic, lime zest, and the remaining oil. Process until well blended, and then add this mixture to the tomatoes.
5. Stir in the chopped sweet yellow pepper, thinly sliced spring onions, cumin, smoked paprika, and salt. Allow the salsa to sit for 1 hour to let the flavors meld.

Nutritional Information (per serving - 1/2 cup): Calories - 36, Protein: 1g, Carbohydrates: 7g, Fat: 1g

Decadent Cranberry Ripe Slice

Ingredients:

- 80g of finely chopped cacao butter

- 1 round tablespoon of coconut oil

- 1 cup of dried cranberries

- 1/2 cup of desiccated coconut

- 1/2 teaspoon of vanilla powder

- 2 tablespoons of agave nectar

Classic Dark Chocolate Topping:

- 60g of finely chopped cacao butter

- 1 tablespoon of coconut oil

- 1/2 teaspoon of vanilla powder

- 1 tablespoon of dark agave nectar

- A pinch of Celtic salt

- 1/3 cup of cacao powder

Instructions:

1. Begin by placing finely chopped cacao butter in a glass bowl. Melt it over a bowl of boiling water. Once melted, remove it from the heat.

2. Whisk in coconut oil, vanilla powder, dark agave nectar, a pinch of Celtic salt, and cacao powder, adding the cacao powder last. Whisk until you have a smooth mixture and set it aside.

3. Chill half of the prepared Classic Dark Chocolate in the base of a lined, sealable glass dish, keeping the other half warm.

4. In a food processor, process dried cranberries, desiccated coconut, vanilla powder, and agave nectar until the mixture becomes fine and begins to bind.

5. Press the cranberry mixture firmly onto the hardened chocolate.

6. Spread the remaining chocolate over the slice and chill until it becomes firm.

7. Once firm, cut into squares and serve this Decadent Cranberry Ripe Slice, which serves 4-6.

Nutritional Information (per serving - 1 square, makes 4-6 servings): Calories - 150, Protein: 1g, Carbohydrates: 15g, Fat: 11g

Nutty Walnut Cookies - A Healthier Twist

Ingredients:

- 2.5 cups of ground walnuts

- 2/3 cup of spelt flour

- 1 teaspoon of salt

- 1/3 cup of ground flaxseed

- 1/2 cup of maple syrup

- 1/2 teaspoon of vanilla extract

Instructions:

1. Begin by mixing all the dry ingredients in a bowl.

2. Add the wet ingredients and mix thoroughly until well combined.

3. Grease a baking tray lightly with oil, then roll the dough into small balls and place them on the tray. Flatten each ball with a fork.

4. Place a walnut on top of each cookie.

5. Bake at 180°C/350°F for 10-15 minutes, or until the cookies are golden brown (be cautious not to let them burn).

6. Allow the cookies to cool on the tray before removing them.

7. This recipe yields about 24 cookies. Enjoy your healthier walnut cookies!

Nutritional Information (per cookie, assuming 24 cookies): Calories - 92, Protein: 2g, Carbohydrates: 6g, Fat: 7g

Fragrant Chai Spice Blend (Chai Latte)

Ingredients:

- 1/3 cup of Ceylon cinnamon, finely ground

- 2 tablespoons of ground cardamom

- 2 tablespoons of ground ginger

- 1 tablespoon of ground cloves

- 1 tablespoon of ground nutmeg

Instructions:

1. Combine all the spices thoroughly and store the blend in an airtight jar.

To make a Chai Latte (serves 1):

1. In a blender, combine 1 cup of coconut milk, 1 medjool date, 1/2 teaspoon of chai spice, a dash of vanilla extract, and a pinch of Celtic salt.

2. Blend until smooth, then transfer the mixture to a small saucepan.

3. Heat to your preferred temperature and enjoy a delightful Chai Latte.

Nutritional Information (per serving, assuming 1 serving of Chai Latte): Calories - 174, Protein: 2g, Carbohydrates: 24g, Fat: 9g

Nutty Tahini Delights

Ingredients:

- 1 cup of spelt flour

- 1/2 tsp of bicarbonate soda

- 1/2 tsp of Celtic salt

- 3/4 cup of tahini

- 3/4 cup of maple syrup

- 1 tsp of vanilla extract

- 1/2 cup of chopped pistachios

- 1/2 cup of chopped dried cranberries

Instructions:

1. Preheat your oven to 190°C/375°F and line a cookie tray with baking paper.

2. In a large bowl, combine the spelt flour, bicarbonate soda, and Celtic salt.

3. Make a well in the center of the dry ingredients, and pour in the tahini and maple syrup.

4. Mix until well combined, resulting in a stiff cookie dough.

5. Scoop out tablespoons of dough and shape them into rounds or squares using wet hands. Place them apart on the cookie tray.

6. Bake for 10 minutes; do not overbake, even if they appear undercooked. Allow them to cool on the tray, then transfer to an airtight container. This recipe yields 18 delightful cookies.

Nutritional Information (per cookie, assuming 18 servings): Calories - 222, Protein: 4g, Carbohydrates: 26g, Fat: 12g

Spiced Ginger Gems

Ingredients:

- 100g of spelt flour

- 2 tsp of ground ginger

- 40g of coconut sugar

- 50g of coconut oil

- 1 level tsp of bicarbonate soda

- 2 tbsp of honey

Instructions:

1. Preheat your oven to 170°C/340°F and line two large baking trays with nonstick baking paper.

2. In a large bowl, sift the spelt flour, ground ginger, and coconut sugar.

3. Make a well in the center and add the melted coconut oil and honey. Stir until the mixture comes together to form a soft dough.

4. Divide the dough into two halves, and then cut each piece into 8 portions.

5. Roll each portion into a ball and place them well apart on the baking trays, then gently flatten them.

6. Bake for 12-14 minutes until they turn golden and develop a cracked appearance on top.

7. Allow the biscuits to firm up on the trays for 10 minutes, and then transfer them to a wire rack to cool completely. Store these delectable spiced ginger gems in an airtight container for up to a week.

Nutritional Information (per cookie, assuming 16 servings): Calories - 150, Protein: 1g, Carbohydrates: 17g, Fat: 9g

Date-Filled Oat Delights

Filling:

- 1 cup of Medjool dates, pitted

- 1/2 apple, cored and diced

- 1/4 cup of maple syrup

- 1/2 tsp of ground cardamom

- 1 tsp of vanilla extract

Dough:

- 3 cups of oat flour

- 1/3 cup of coconut sugar

- 2 tsp of baking powder

- 1/2 tsp of Celtic salt

- 2 tsp of vanilla extract

- 1 cup of water

Glaze:

- 1/2 cup of coconut sugar (powdered in a food processor or thermomix)

- 2 tbsp of boiling water

- 1/2 tsp of vanilla extract

Instructions:

1. Preheat your oven to 180°C (375°F) and line a baking sheet while spraying it with oil.

2. Prepare the filling by processing the Medjool dates, diced apple, maple syrup, ground cardamom, and vanilla extract in a food processor or blender until smooth. Set it aside.

3. For the dough, combine the dry ingredients in a large bowl and mix well. Then, mix the vanilla extract and water together.

4. While stirring, pour the wet mixture into the dry ingredients and continue mixing until a dough forms. Note that this is not a very wet dough but should be slightly sticky.

5. Turn the dough out onto a sheet of baking paper and shape it into a rectangle. Place another sheet of baking paper on top.

6. Roll the dough into a 1cm (1/4in) thick layer. Remove the top layer of baking paper and discard it.

7. Spread the prepared filling evenly over the dough.

8. Starting from one shorter end, roll up the dough, then cut it into 8 pieces.

9. Place the cut side up onto the prepared baking sheet.

10. Bake for 20-25 minutes or until the rolls are set but not overly dry. Remove them from the oven and allow them to cool slightly.

11. While the rolls are still warm, drizzle them with the glaze. Store them in an airtight container for up to 2 days. Enjoy this delightful treat.

Nutritional information: Protein: Approximately 2-4g per serving (assuming 8 servings), Carbohydrates: Approximately 40-50g per serving, Fat: Approximately 4-6g per serving

Sultana Cookies

Ingredients:

- 3/4 cup of coconut sugar

- 1/4 cup + 3 tablespoons of unsweetened almond milk

- 1/4 cup + 2 tablespoons of smooth nut butter

- 1 2/3 cups of spelt flour

- 1/2 tsp of baking soda

- 1/2 cup of sultanas

Instructions:

1. Preheat the oven to 190°C (360°F).

2. In a large bowl, mix the sugar and almond milk until the sugar dissolves completely. Add the nut butter and stir until well combined.

3. Add the dry ingredients, being careful not to over-mix to avoid making the cookies gummy.

4. Gently fold in the sultanas until they are evenly distributed.

5. Scoop heaping tablespoons of cookie dough onto a non-stick baking sheet, leaving some space between them as the cookies will spread while baking.

6. Bake the cookies for 14-16 minutes, depending on your desired level of crunchiness.

7. Remove the cookies from the oven and transfer them to cooling racks for 5-10 minutes.

Nutritional Information per cookie: Calories - 115, Fat: 4g, Carbohydrates: 18g, Fiber: 2g, Protein: 3g

Almond Pulp Cookies

This recipe is a great way to use up almond pulp left over from making almond milk.

Ingredients:

- 1 cup wet almond pulp

- 1 cup shredded coconut

- 1/3 cup maple syrup

- 1 flax egg

- 1/2 cup chopped cranberries

Instructions:

1. Preheat your oven to 350°F (180°C).

2. Mix all the ingredients in a medium bowl.

3. Cover a cookie sheet with parchment paper, lightly greased with oil spray.

4. Scoop the dough with a spoon and place it on the sheet, then press down on top.

5. Bake for about 20 minutes or until golden brown.

6. Makes approximately 12 cookies.

Nutritional Information (per serving - 1 cookie): Calories - 110, Fat: 4g, Carbohydrates: 19g, Fiber: 2g, Protein: 2g

Corn and Black Bean Salsa

Ingredients:

- 4 ears of corn, cooked and kernels cut off

- 2 cans black beans, washed and drained

- 1/2 cup finely chopped red onion

- 1/2 cup spring onions, chopped

- 1/2 cup fresh coriander/cilantro, chopped

- 2 cups cherry/grape tomatoes, quartered

Dressing:

- 1/2 cup olive oil

- 4 tbsp lime juice

- 1 tbsp lemon juice

- 1 tsp cumin

- 1 garlic clove, crushed

- 1 tsp Celtic salt

Instructions:

1. Place chopped ingredients in a large bowl.

2. Place all dressing ingredients in a jar and shake well.

3. Pour over vegetables and mix well.

Nutritional Information (per serving): Calories - 260, Fat: 15g, Carbohydrates: 31g, Fiber: 9g, Protein: 9g

Savory Almond Pulp Crackers

Ingredients:

- 1 cup wet almond pulp (leftover from making almond milk)

- 3 tbsp olive or coconut oil

- 1 tbsp ground flaxseeds

- 1/4 tsp Celtic salt

- 1 garlic clove, minced

- Water as needed

- 2 tsp dried herbs (such as chives, rosemary, or parsley)

Instructions:

1. Preheat the oven to 180°C/350°F.

2. In a large mixing bowl, combine the dry ingredients and stir well.

3. If the dough appears dry, add water one tablespoon at a time until it can be easily pressed together.

4. Place the mixture between two sheets of parchment paper and roll it out to your desired thickness.

5. Use a knife to score the rolled dough into square shapes, making about 20 crackers. Poke the middle of each cracker with a fork to help them bake evenly.

6. Transfer the parchment paper with the cut crackers to a baking sheet.

7. Bake for 10 minutes, then flip each cracker and bake until they become crisp and golden, which should take about 10 more minutes.

8. Allow the crackers to cool completely before serving. They can be stored at room temperature for a few days or in the fridge for an extended shelf life. This recipe makes approximately 20 crackers.

Nutritional Information (per serving - 5 crackers): Calories - 110, Fat: 8g, Carbohydrates: 8g, Fiber: 3g, Protein: 3g

Gluten-Free Buckwheat Sourdough Bread

Ingredients:

- 2 tsp salt

- 3 1/2 cups water

- 1 to 2 cups of buckwheat starter (bring it to room temperature if stored in the fridge)

- 2 cups millet flour

- 2 cups quinoa flour (or sorghum flour)

- 2 cups buckwheat flour

- 1/4 cup psyllium husk

- 2 tbsp olive oil

Instructions:

1. In a bowl, combine salt, water, and the buckwheat starter, mixing well to dissolve the salt.

2. Add the various flours and olive oil, mixing thoroughly. Add the psyllium husk last, ensuring it's well incorporated. The dough should resemble a very thick cake batter. You may need to adjust the water or flour to get the right consistency.

3. Place the dough in a well-oiled bread tin. You can optionally sprinkle sesame seeds both in the tin and on top of the bread, which has also been lightly oiled. Cover with a lid or plastic wrap.

4. Allow the dough to rise for 3-4 hours, depending on room temperature. The dough should expand by a third to half its original size.

5. Bake at 180°C for 1 1/2 hours. You can cover the bread tin with foil during the first hour to prevent drying out or over-browning.

6. Once baked, remove from the tin and let the bread cool on a rack. For the easiest slicing, wait until the bread is cold.

Nutritional Information (per serving - 1 slice): Calories - 180, Fat: 2g, Carbohydrates: 38g, Fiber: 6g, Protein: 5g

Crispy Cauliflower Wings

Ingredients:

- 550g cauliflower florets

- 3 tbsp tomato paste

- 1 tsp minced garlic

- 1/4 tsp cayenne pepper

- 1/3 cup soy sauce

- 2 tbsp maple syrup

- 2 tbsp fresh lime juice

Instructions:

1. Preheat your oven to 230°C (450°F) and line a baking sheet with parchment paper or a silicone baking mat. Also, heat a large nonstick pan over medium heat.

2. In a large mixing bowl, combine all the sauce ingredients. Add the cauliflower and toss until it is evenly coated.

3. Once the pan is hot, add the cauliflower (using a slotted spoon to leave the excess marinade behind). Keep the remaining marinade.

4. Cook the cauliflower, stirring frequently, until it browns and most of the liquid has evaporated, about 10 minutes.

5. Remove the cauliflower from the pan, place it on the prepared baking sheet, and pour some of the leftover marinade over it. Roast the cauliflower in the oven for 20 minutes.

6. Serve the cauliflower with rice. This recipe serves 4.

Nutritional Information (per serving): Calories - 150, Fat: 1g, Carbohydrates: 30g, Fiber: 4g, Protein: 5g

Gluten-Free Buckwheat Seed Bread

Ingredients:

- 500g hulled buckwheat kernels

- 200ml water

- 1/4 tsp Celtic salt

- 2 tsp poppy seeds and pepitas (or seeds of your choice)

Instructions:

1. Rinse the buckwheat thoroughly and transfer it to a large bowl. Cover it with cold water and a cloth. Let it soak overnight.

2. Drain (do not rinse) and transfer to a blender with 200ml of water and salt. Blend, starting at low speed and slowly increasing.

3. Transfer the mixture back to the bowl and allow it to sit covered at room temperature for 24 hours.

4. Preheat the oven to 180°C (350°F).

5. Line a loaf pan with baking paper and transfer the dough into it. Sprinkle with your choice of seeds.

6. Bake for 90 minutes. Allow it to cool before slicing and enjoying.

7. The bread can be stored in a sealed container for 4-5 days. If you won't consume it all during this time, slice it and freeze the portions for up to a month. This way, you can toast a slice whenever you want delicious bread.

Nutritional Information (per slice): Calories - 70, Fat: 1g, Carbohydrates: 14g, Fiber: 2g, Protein: 3g

Vegan Tofu Cottage Cheese

Ingredients:

- 450g firm tofu, drained

- 1 1/4 tbsp fresh chives, minced

- 1 tsp fresh parsley, minced

- 1/4 tsp dill weed

- 1/4 cup water

- 1 tsp Celtic salt

- 1.5 tsp fresh lemon juice

- 1 tsp each onion & garlic powder

Instructions:

1. Begin by mashing the tofu, then reserve 1/2 cup of mashed tofu.

2. Combine the tofu with chives, parsley, and dill.

3. Process the reserved tofu until it becomes smooth.

4. Combine all the ingredients, including the smooth tofu, and mix thoroughly.

5. Refrigerate until the flavors blend.

6. This recipe serves 4.

Nutritional Information (per serving): Calories - 105, Fat: 5g, Carbohydrates: 3g, Fiber: 1g, Protein: 10g

Homemade Seed Crackers

Ingredients:

- 1 cup pumpkin seeds

- 1/3 cup sunflower seeds

- 1/4 cup sesame seeds

- 3/4 cup ground flaxseed

- 1 tsp Celtic salt

- 1/2 tsp ginger powder

- 1 tsp garlic powder

- Cayenne pepper to taste

- 1 tbsp chopped fresh or dried rosemary

- 1.5 cups boiling water

Instructions:

1. Combine all the dry ingredients in a bowl.

2. Pour the boiling water over the dry ingredients and stir. Allow it to sit for a few minutes until it clumps together.

3. Spread the mixture over an oven tray (the thinner, the crunchier).

4. Bake at 190°C (375°F) for 40 minutes.

5. Allow to cool, break it into pieces, and store in an airtight container.

Nutritional Information (per 1 oz serving - about 5 crackers): Calories - 150, Fat: 12g, Carbohydrates: 8g, Fiber: 5g, Protein: 6g

Oil-Free Hummus

Ingredients:

- 1 1/2 cups cooked chickpeas

- 1/2 cup aquafaba (cooking water from chickpeas)

- 1/4 cup fresh lemon juice

- 3-4 tbsp water

- 1/2 cup organic tahini

- 1-2 garlic cloves

- 1/8 - 1/4 tsp Celtic salt

Instructions:

1. Blend all the ingredients in a food processor or high-speed blender until smooth and creamy.

2. Spoon the hummus into a bowl and sprinkle with sumac, black sesame seeds, and lemon juice.

3. Cover and store the hummus in the fridge.

4. Serve it cold with fresh carrot and celery sticks or use it as a dressing.

5. Leftover hummus keeps well in the refrigerator, covered, for up to 1 week.

Nutritional Information (per 2 oz serving): Calories - 50, Fat: 3g, Carbohydrates: 5g, Protein: 2g

Strawberry Oat Cookies

Ingredients:

- 2 large ripe bananas, mashed (⅔ cup)

- 1/4 cup maple syrup

- 2/3 cup almond butter

- 2 cups rolled oats

- 1/2 tsp Celtic salt

- 3/4 cup fresh strawberries, chopped into chunks

- 1 tsp vanilla extract

Instructions:

1. Preheat the oven to 180°F (350°C) and line a large baking sheet.

2. In a large bowl, combine the mashed bananas, maple syrup, almond butter, and vanilla until well blended.

3. Add the rolled oats and salt, mixing well.

4. Stir in the fresh strawberry chunks until they are evenly distributed in the cookie dough.

5. Drop spoonfuls of the dough onto the prepared baking sheet.

6. Bake the cookies on the center rack of the preheated oven for 10-15 minutes, until the edges are slightly golden and they feel firm when touched.

7. Allow the cookies to cool for at least 10 minutes.

Nutritional Information (per serving - 2 cookies): Calories - 190, Fat: 8g, Carbohydrates: 26g, Fiber: 3g, Protein: 4g

Mexican Cashew Cheese Dip

Ingredients:

- 1 cup raw cashews

- 1/2 cup water

- 2 tbsp lemon juice

- 2 tsp miso

- 1/2 tsp garlic powder

- 1 tsp smoked paprika

- 1 1/4 cups chopped tomatoes

- Celtic salt to taste

- Pinch of cayenne pepper

Instructions:

1. Boil the raw cashews for 5 minutes or soak them in hot water for 30 minutes. Drain the cashews and transfer them to a high-speed blender.

2. Add all the ingredients to the blender along with half of the chopped tomatoes.

3. Blend until the mixture is smooth and creamy.

4. Transfer the cheese sauce to a saucepan and add the remaining tomatoes. Cook until it thickens.

5. Pour the dip into a serving bowl and enjoy with chips or as a sandwich spread. This dip serves 6-8.

Nutritional Information (per serving): Calories - 120, Fat: 8g, Carbohydrates: 8g, Protein: 4g

Delicious Almond Butter Squares

Ingredients:

- 1/2 cup coconut sugar

- 1 cup almond butter

- 1 tsp vanilla extract

- 3/4 cup spelt flour

- 1/4 cup chickpea flour

- 1 tsp bicarbonate soda

- 1/2 tsp baking powder

- 1/2 cup soy milk

- 1 cup rolled oats

- 1/2 cup chopped almonds

- 1/2 cup medjool dates, pitted and chopped

Instructions:

1. Preheat your oven to 180°C (350°F) and grease and line an 8-inch square baking tin.

2. In a mixing bowl, use a hand or stand mixer to blend coconut sugar and almond butter on medium speed for about 5 minutes.

3. Mix in vanilla extract.

4. Add spelt flour, chickpea flour, bicarbonate soda, and baking powder, then mix on medium speed.

5. Stir in rolled oats and mix briefly until combined.

6. Fold in chopped almonds and dates.

7. Use your hands to press the dough lightly into the prepared dish.

8. Bake for 15 to 20 minutes, or until it's lightly golden brown.

9. Allow it to cool on a wire rack before cutting into sixteen squares.

Nutritional Information (per serving): Calories - 240, Fat: 12g, Carbohydrates: 28g, Protein: 6g

Moroccan Spiced Carrot Dip

Ingredients:

- 500g carrots

- 2 tbsp olive oil

- 2 garlic cloves

- 1/2 tsp ground cumin

- 1/2 tsp sweet paprika

- 1/2 tsp ground ginger

- 1/2 tsp ground cardamom

- 1/2 tsp Celtic salt

- 1/2 tsp honey

- 2 tsp lemon juice

- 2 tbsp flat-leaf parsley

Instructions:

1. Peel the carrots and cut them into chunks. Cook them in salted water for about 20 minutes until they are soft. Drain and return them to the pan to cook for an additional 2 minutes to dry out the carrots.

2. Transfer the carrots and garlic to a food processor. Add the remaining ingredients and process until smooth.

3. This recipe serves 4-6.

Nutritional Information (per serving): Calories - 95, Fat: 4g, Carbohydrates: 14g, Protein: 2g

Creamy Almond Cheese

Ingredients:

- 1 1/4 cups almonds, pre-soaked and peeled

- 1/4 cup lemon juice

- 1/2 cup water

- 2 tbsp olive oil

- 2 cloves garlic, minced

- 1 1/8 tsp Celtic salt

Instructions:

1. Soak the almonds for at least 8 hours or overnight. After soaking, rinse and peel them.

2. Transfer the soaked and peeled almonds to a blender, add the lemon juice, water, olive oil, minced garlic, and Celtic salt.

3. Blend the mixture until it becomes smooth.

4. Pour the mixture into a cheese cloth and tie it with a rubber band. Allow it to sit for 2-3 hours or overnight.

5. Once drained, scoop the creamy almond cheese into a container.

6. Store it in the fridge, and it will keep well for about a week.

7. This recipe serves 6.

Nutritional Information (per serving - 1/4 cup): Calories - 238, Fat: 21g, Carbohydrates: 8g, Protein: 7g

DRESSING-SAUCES-CONDIMENTS

Creamy Avocado Salad Dressing

Ingredients:
- 1 medium avocado
- Juice of one lemon
- 8 tablespoons of olive oil
- 1/2 teaspoon of maple syrup
- 1 teaspoon of Celtic salt
- 2 small cloves of garlic
- 1/3 cup of water

Instructions:
1. Blend all the ingredients until smooth. Pour the dressing over your salad just before serving.
2. Store any leftover dressing in the fridge; it will keep for up to 4 days.

Nutritional Information (per 2 tablespoons): Calories - 90, Protein: 1g, Carbohydrates: 3g, Fat: 9g

Vegan Worcestershire-Style Sauce

Ingredients:
- 1/2 cup of lemon juice
- 1/4 cup of water
- 2 tablespoons of coconut sugar
- 2 tablespoons of maple syrup
- 3 tablespoons of soy sauce
- 1/2 teaspoon of onion powder
- 1/2 teaspoon of garlic powder
- 1/4 teaspoon of Ceylon cinnamon

Instructions:
1. In a saucepan, combine lemon juice, water, coconut sugar, maple syrup, soy sauce, onion powder, garlic powder, and cinnamon. Heat over medium heat.

2. Whisk the sauce while heating to dissolve the sugar and mix it thoroughly. Bring it to a simmer and then turn off the heat. Let it cool completely.

3. Transfer the sauce to an airtight container and refrigerate. It will stay fresh for up to 2 months in the fridge.

Nutritional Information (per 1 tablespoon): Calories - 13, Protein: 0g, Carbohydrates: 3g, Fat: 0g

Zesty Italian Vinaigrette

Ingredients:
- 1/2 cup of olive oil
- 1/4 cup of lemon juice
- 1/2 teaspoon of maple syrup
- 1/2 cup of water
- 1 small clove of garlic
- 1.5 teaspoons of dried marjoram
- 1.5 teaspoons of oregano
- 1.5 teaspoons of dried basil
- 1.5 teaspoons of Celtic salt

Instructions:
1. In a blender, combine olive oil, water, lemon juice, maple syrup, and garlic until a smooth mixture forms.
2. Add the remaining ingredients and blend briefly.
3. Store in the refrigerator, and it will keep well for up to 5 days.

Nutritional Information (per serving - 2 tablespoons): Calories - 72, Protein: 0g, Carbohydrates: 2g, Fat: 7g

Creamy Almond Dressing

Yield: 1/2 cup
Ingredients:
- 1/4 cup of raw almonds
- 2 teaspoons of 'mustard'
- 2 small cloves of garlic
- Juice of 1 lemon
- 2 tablespoons of soy sauce
- 1/2 teaspoon of miso paste

- 1 tablespoon of flax seeds
- 1/3 cup of water

Instructions:
1. Place all the ingredients in a blender and blend until the mixture is smooth.
2. Store the dressing in an airtight container, and it will stay fresh for up to a week.

Nutritional Information (per 2 tablespoons): Calories - 47, Protein: 1g, Carbohydrates: 3g, Fat: 4g

Fresh Herb Curry Paste

Ingredients:
- 2 large cloves of garlic, finely minced
- 1 tablespoon of fresh ginger, finely grated
- 1 cup of fresh coriander leaves
- 1 cup of fresh mint leaves
- 1 cup of fresh basil leaves
- 1/4 to 1/2 cup of water (adjust for desired consistency)

Instructions:
1. Begin by finely mincing the two large garlic cloves and grating the fresh ginger.
2. In a food processor, combine the minced garlic, grated ginger, fresh coriander leaves, mint leaves, and basil leaves.
3. Gradually add 1/4 to 1/2 cup of water to achieve the desired paste consistency.
4. Process until you have a smooth and aromatic Fresh Herb Curry Paste.

Nutritional Information (per serving - 2 tablespoons): Calories - 10, Protein: 0.5g, Carbohydrates: 2g, Fat: 0g

Creamy Garlic Butter Spread

Yield: 2 cups

Ingredients:

- 1 cup of water

- 1/2 cup of raw cashews

- 4 teaspoons of lemon juice

- 3 cloves of garlic

- 1/4 teaspoon of miso paste

- 1 teaspoon of onion powder

- 1 teaspoon of Celtic salt

- 1/2 teaspoon of dried dill

- 3/4 cup of warm, cooked cornmeal

Instructions:

1. In a high-speed blender, process the raw cashews with half of the water until you achieve a very smooth consistency.

2. Drizzle in the remaining water and add the lemon juice, garlic cloves, miso paste, onion powder, Celtic salt, and dried dill. Continue blending until the mixture is very smooth.

3. Store the Creamy Garlic Butter Spread in an airtight container in the refrigerator.

Serving Suggestions:

1. For garlic bread, spread the Garlic Butter on sliced bread and bake at 180°C (350°F) for approximately 10-15 minutes.

2. For pasta, cook pasta according to package instructions, drain, return it to the pot, and stir in enough Garlic Butter to coat. Heat through.

Nutritional Information (per 2 tablespoons): Calories - 35, Protein: 1g, Carbohydrates: 3g, Fat: 2g

Creamy Almond Mayo

Yield: 2 cups

Ingredients:

- 2 cups of water

- 1/2 cup of blanched almonds

- 1 teaspoon of agar agar

- 1/2 tablespoon of lemon juice

- 1/2 teaspoon of onion powder

- 1/2 teaspoon of Celtic salt

- 1/4 teaspoon of garlic powder

Instructions:

1. Process half of the water with the blanched almonds, strain, and save the liquid (you can use the almond pulp in patties or waffles).

2. In a small saucepan, cook the remaining water with agar agar until it's almost boiled. Remove it from heat.

3. Pour everything into a high-speed blender and blend until smooth.

4. Transfer the creamy mixture into a jar and refrigerate.

Nutritional Information (per 2 tablespoons): Calories - 37, Protein: 1g, Carbohydrates: 2g, Fat: 3g

Homemade Almond Mustard

Yield: 2/3 cup

Ingredients:

- 1/2 cup of almond mayonnaise

- 1 tablespoon of finely chopped parsley

- 2 teaspoons of lemon juice

- 1 teaspoon of grated onion

- 1 teaspoon of turmeric powder

- 1/8 teaspoon of garlic powder

- 1/8 teaspoon of onion powder

- 1/8 teaspoon of paprika

- 1/4 teaspoon of Celtic salt

Instructions:

1. Process all the ingredients in a high-speed blender until well combined.

2. Keep the Homemade Almond Mustard refrigerated in an airtight container.

Nutritional Information (per 1 tablespoon): Calories - 13, Protein: 0g, Carbohydrates: 0g, Fat: 1g

Fresh Basil Pesto Without Nuts

Ingredients (Serves 8):

- 2 cups of fresh basil leaves, firmly packed

- 1 clove of garlic, finely chopped

- 1 teaspoon of finely grated lemon zest

- 2 tablespoons of lightly toasted sunflower seeds

- 2 tablespoons of lightly toasted pumpkin seeds

- 2 tablespoons of olive oil

- 1/4 cup of water

Instructions:

1. In a food processor, combine basil, garlic, lemon zest, and the toasted seeds. Pulse until the mixture is roughly chopped.

2. With the food processor running, gradually add the olive oil and water until the mixture is well combined and reaches a thick, pesto-like consistency.

3. This nut-free basil pesto can be used as a flavorful base in pasta dishes, with beans, or as a spread.

Nutritional Information (per serving, serving size may vary): Calories - 65, Protein: 1g, Carbohydrates: 1g, Fat: 6g

Homemade Seasoning Blend

Ingredients:

- 5 tablespoons of Celtic salt

- 2 tablespoons of garlic powder

- 1.5 tablespoons of oregano

- 1/2 teaspoon of turmeric

- 1/4 teaspoon of celery salt

- 1.5 tablespoons of basil

- 5 tablespoons of dried parsley

- 2 tablespoons of paprika

- 1.5 tablespoons of onion powder

Instructions:

Blend all the ingredients in a dry blender until it becomes a fine powder. Seal the seasoning in a jar and store it in the pantry.

Nutritional Information (per teaspoon): Calories - 7, Fat: 0g, Carbohydrates: 2g, Fiber: 1g, Protein: 0g

Homemade Tomato

Ingredients:

- 1/2 cup tomato paste

- 1/2 cup water

- 1 1/2 tbsp lemon juice

- 1/2 tsp garlic powder

- 1 tbsp maple syrup

- 1/2 tsp onion powder

- 1/2 tsp Celtic salt

Instructions:

1. In a saucepan, combine the carefully measured ingredients. Whisk them together well.

2. Turn on the heat and cook the mixture until it starts to bubble, approximately 4 minutes, stirring constantly.

3. Remove from heat and store in a glass jar in the refrigerator.

4. This recipe yields 1 cup and can be stored in the fridge for 2-3 weeks when well ealed.

Nutritional Information (per 2 tbsp serving): Calories - 35, Fat: 0g, Carbohydrates: 9g, Sugar: 5g, Protein: 0g

Smoky Bbq Sauce

Ingredients:

- 1 1/4 cups tomato ketchup

- 4 tbsp lemon juice

- 5 tbsp rapadura sugar

- 2 tbsp molasses

- 3 tbsp honey

- 2 tbsp oil

- 1.5 tsp smoked paprika

- Celtic salt to taste

- 1 tbsp Worcestershire sauce

Instructions:

1. In a saucepan, combine all the ingredients and mix thoroughly.

2. Heat the mixture over medium-high heat until it begins to boil, then simmer for 5 minutes.

3. Turn off the heat and allow it to cool before serving or storing.

4. This recipe yields 2 cups and can be stored in the fridge for up to 3 weeks.

Nutritional Information (per 2 tbsp serving): Calories - 60, Fat: 2g, Carbohydrates: 12g, Sugar: 11g, Protein: 0g

Homemade Golden Spread

Ingredients:

- 250g copha, chopped (vegetable shortening)

- 240g light olive oil

- 160ml water

- 3g turmeric

- 5g Celtic salt

Instructions:

1. Blend or process the ingredients until the mixture is smooth and creamy, similar to margarine. It will thicken up a little more as it stands.

2. Use this spread to replace butter or margarine in recipes.

3. Store the spread in the fridge for up to 2 weeks. You can also cut it in half and store the second half in the freezer for up to 3 months.

Nutritional Information (per 1 tbsp serving): Calories - 80, Fat: 9g, Carbohydrates: 0g, Protein: 0g

Asian-Style Salad Dressing

Ingredients:

- 1/4 cup tahini

- 1 tbsp honey

- 1/4 cup + 2 tbsp coconut aminos

- 1/4 cup + 2 tbsp green onions

- 1.5 tbsp sesame oil

- 1/2 cup of water

- 1/4 tsp cumin

- Celtic salt, to taste

- 1.5 tbsp olive oil

- 1.5 cloves of garlic

- 1.5 tbsp chopped ginger

Instructions:

1. In a blender, combine all the ingredients listed above and blend until you achieve a smooth consistency.

2. Chill the dressing in the refrigerator before serving.

3. Serve this dressing over your favorite salad.

4. It can be stored in the fridge for up to 2 weeks.

5. This dressing recipe serves 10.

Nutritional Information (per serving): Calories - 95, Fat: 8g, Carbohydrates: 6g, Protein: 2g

Cashew Parmesan

Ingredients:

- 1/2 cup raw cashews

- 1/2 tsp garlic powder

- 1/2 tsp stock powder

- 1/2 tsp Celtic salt

Instructions:

1. Combine all the ingredients and pulse until they resemble the texture of Parmesan cheese.

2. Store the cashew Parmesan in an airtight container in the refrigerator for up to 6 weeks.

3. This recipe yields 2/3 cup, and a serving size is approximately 1 teaspoon.

Nutritional Information (per serving): Calories - 9, Fat: 1g, Carbohydrates: 1g, Protein: 0g

Sage Gravy

Ingredients:

- 2 tbsp fresh sage, sliced

- 1 sliced shallot

- 2 tbsp stock powder

- 2 cups water

- 1/4 cup cold water

- 3 tbsp cornflour

- Celtic salt to taste

Instructions:

1. Heat the sage and shallot with a small amount of water and cook until they become tender.

2. Add the stock and 2 cups of water, then bring to a boil.

3. Create a slurry by mixing the cornflour with 1/4 cup of cold water and add it to the broth to allow it to thicken.

4. Remove from heat.

5. This recipe serves 9.

Nutritional Information (per serving): Calories - 20, Fat: 0g, Carbohydrates: 4g, Protein: 1g

Mushroom Gravy

Ingredients:

- 450g mushrooms, sliced

- 1/2 tsp garlic powder

- 1/2 tsp stock powder

- 1/2 tsp onion powder

- 2 cups almond milk

- 1/2 tsp Celtic salt

- 1 tsp lemon juice

Instructions:

1. Sauté the sliced mushrooms with a small amount of water over medium heat until they become tender.

2. Transfer the cooked mushrooms and the remaining ingredients to a blender.

3. Blend until the mixture is smooth.

4. This recipe serves 6.

Nutritional Information (per serving): Calories - 30, Fat: 1g, Carbohydrates: 4g, Protein: 2g

Fresh Basil Pesto

Ingredients:

- 2 cups fresh basil

- 1/4 cup toasted pine nuts

- 1/4 cup olive oil

- 2 garlic cloves

- 1/2 tsp Celtic salt

- 1/4 cup lemon juice

Instructions:

1. Place all the ingredients in a food processor and pulse until the mixture becomes smooth.

2. Store the fresh basil pesto in a jar in the fridge; it will keep well for a week.

3. For an extra boost of omega-3s, consider adding a few walnuts.

Nutritional Information (per serving - 2 tbsp): Calories - 88, Fat: 9g, Carbohydrates: 2g, Protein: 1g

Dairy-Free Cheese Sauce

Ingredients:

- 2 cups potatoes, peeled and roughly chopped

- 1 cup peeled carrots, diced

- 1/4 of a small-sized onion, roughly chopped

- 2 tbsp miso

- 1 tbsp lemon juice

- 1 tsp garlic powder

- 1 tsp onion powder

- 1/2 tsp Celtic salt

- 1/2 – 3/4 cup warm water

Instructions:

1. Boil the potatoes, carrots, and onion until they are soft, usually taking 15-20 minutes. Drain them once they are done and add them to your blender.

2. Place all the remaining ingredients into your blender and blend until the cheese sauce is smooth and creamy. If it's too thick, you can add a little more water while blending. You shouldn't need to heat it up on the stove as the veggies will still be hot.

3. Pour the cheese sauce into a bowl and enjoy. Store any leftovers in an airtight container in the fridge for up to a week.

Nutritional Information (per serving): Calories - 110, Fat: 1g, Carbohydrates: 23g, Fiber: 5g, Protein: 3g

DESSERTS

Minty Nutty Dessert Bars

Ingredients:

Base:

- 1 cup of macadamia nuts or almonds (or a mix of both)

- 1/2 cup of dates

Peppermint Filling:

- 1 cup of cashews

- 5-8 drops of peppermint essential oil

- 1/4 cup of coconut cream

- 1/4 cup of sweetener (maple syrup, agave, or honey)

Topping:

- 1/4 cup of carob powder (or a blend of 1/2 carob and 1/2 cacao powder)

- 1/4 cup of sweetener

- 1/3 cup of coconut oil

- 1/4 cup of hazelnuts (or cashews)

- 1/2 teaspoon of vanilla extract

Instructions:

Base:

1. Process nuts and dates in a food processor. Add a tiny amount of water only if necessary.

2. Press the mixture into an 8x10" shallow dish using wet hands.

Peppermint Filling:

1. Begin by blending the cashews until they reach a creamy consistency.

2. Add the peppermint essential oil, coconut cream, and sweetener. Blend until the mixture reaches the right consistency, adding a little water if needed.

3. Spread the filling over the base and then place it in the freezer while making the topping.

Topping:

1. Blend all the topping ingredients in a blender, starting with the nuts. Add a little water as needed to reach a thick paste consistency.

2. Smooth the topping over the set filling and return it to the freezer for 4-6 hours.

Note: You can substitute cashews for hazelnuts.

Nutritional Information (per serving - 1 bar): Calories - 110, Protein: 2g, Carbohydrates: 7g, Fat: 9g

Vegan Carrot Cake

Ingredients:

- 2 tablespoons of milled flaxseed

- 120ml of coconut oil

- 1 tablespoon of lemon juice

- 2 tablespoons of oat milk

- 2 teaspoons of vanilla extract

- 2 large carrots, grated

- 200g of coconut sugar

- 1/2 teaspoon of Celtic salt

- 250g of spelt flour

- 1 3/4 teaspoons of baking powder

- 1/2 teaspoon of bicarbonate soda

- 1 teaspoon of Ceylon cinnamon

- 1/2 teaspoon of nutmeg

- 50g of chopped walnuts

Frosting:

- 300g of vegan cream cheese

- Zest of 2 limes and juice to get 2 1/2 tablespoons

- 90g of coconut sugar

- Extra chopped walnuts

Instructions:

1. Preheat the oven to 200°C (180°C fan)/390°F and line a 23cm springform cake tin with baking paper.

2. In a large bowl, stir milled flaxseeds into 4 tablespoons (60ml) of warm water and set aside for five minutes. Then add coconut oil, lemon juice, oat milk, vanilla extract, grated carrots, coconut sugar, and Celtic salt. Mix well and set aside.

3. In another large bowl, whisk together spelt flour, baking powder, bicarbonate soda, spices, and chopped walnuts.

4. Add the wet ingredients to the dry and mix thoroughly, even if the batter seems dry or stiff.

5. Spoon the mixture evenly into the prepared baking tin and level it out. Bake for about 35 minutes or until a skewer comes out clean.

6. Let the cake cool completely before removing it from the tin.

7. Just before serving, prepare the frosting by mixing vegan cream cheese, lime juice, lime zest, and coconut sugar until smooth and creamy.

8. Spread the frosting on top of the cooled cake and sprinkle with extra chopped walnuts. Slice and serve.

Nutritional Information (per serving - 1 slice, makes 10 servings): Calories - 415, Protein: 6g, Carbohydrates: 52g, Fat: 21g

Decadent Sweet Potato Chocolate Brownies

Ingredients:

- 1/2 cup of pureed sweet potato

- 1/3 cup of honey, maple syrup, or rice malt syrup

- 1/4 cup of coconut oil

- 1/2 cup of self-raising spelt flour

- 1 teaspoon of vanilla extract

- 1/3 cup of cacao powder

- 1/4 teaspoon of baking soda

- 1/2 teaspoon of cayenne pepper (adjust to your spice preference)

- A pinch of Celtic salt

- 3 tablespoons of chia seeds mixed with 6 tablespoons of water (to replace 3 eggs)

- 3/4 cup of chopped nuts (Brazil nuts, cashews, macadamia nuts)

Instructions:

1. Combine pureed sweet potato, honey (or syrup), coconut oil, spelt flour, vanilla, cacao powder, baking soda, cayenne pepper, and Celtic salt.

2. Substitute eggs with chia seeds and water mixture, let it sit for 5 minutes before adding to the mixture.

3. Add the chopped nuts and mix until well combined.

4. Transfer the mixture into a baking dish and bake in the oven at 160°C (320°F) for 30-40 minutes or until it's fully baked.

5. You can adjust the chia/water ratio or use banana to achieve your desired moisture level. Feel free to experiment.

Nutritional Information (per brownie, assuming 12 servings): Calories - 198, Protein: 4g, Carbohydrates: 21g, Fat: 12g

Tropical Ambrosia Delight

Ingredients:

- 2 cups of fresh pineapple chunks

- 2-4 mandarin oranges

- 1 tsp of pure vanilla extract

- 1/4 cup of frozen pineapple juice concentrate

- 3 tablespoons of white or black chia seeds

- 1 tablespoon of honey (optional)

- 2 cups of red seedless grapes, sliced in half

- 1 can (15 oz.) of organic coconut milk

Instructions:

1. In a bowl, mix the coconut milk with pineapple juice, honey (if using), and vanilla.

2. Add the chia seeds and whisk until they are well mixed in, forming a smooth, lump-free mixture. Repeat this process every 5 minutes a few times.

3. Set this "sauce" aside for 2-4 hours or overnight.

4. Prepare the fruits by cutting the pineapple into bite-size chunks, halving the grapes, and cutting each section of the mandarin oranges into halves or thirds.

5. Combine the prepared fruits with the coconut-chia sauce.

6. Serve your ambrosia in a beautiful glass dish. Optionally, top it with fresh raspberries or add strawberries to add more color.

Variation: You can substitute low glycemic fruits like kiwis and berries if preferred. Enjoy your delicious ambrosia!

Nutritional Information (per serving, assuming 6 servings): Calories - 340, Protein: 5g, Carbohydrates: 53g, Fat: 14g

Decadent Dessert Platter

Ingredients:

- 1/3 cup of unrefined coconut oil

- 2 tablespoons of carob (or cacao as a great alternative)

- 3 tablespoons of honey or rice malt syrup (adjust to taste)

- Toppings of your choice: frozen raspberries, almonds, pepitas, and coconut

Instructions:

1. In a pot, melt together unrefined coconut oil, carob (or cacao), and honey (or rice malt syrup) until well combined.

2. Spread this luscious mixture over your chosen toppings, such as frozen raspberries, almonds, pepitas, and coconut.

3. Place the dessert plate in the freezer for at least 30 minutes or until it sets. Avoid the temptation to eat it all at once, as it's a delightful treat.

Nutritional Information (per serving, serving size may vary): Calories - 185, Protein: 2g, Carbohydrates: 13g, Fat: 14g

Silken Tofu Delight Cheesecake

Ingredients:

Base:

- 1 cup of desiccated coconut

- 1/2 cup of spelt flour

- 1/2 cup of blended nuts

- 1/4 tsp of Celtic salt

- 1/4 cup of maple syrup

- 1/4 cup of coconut oil

Filling:

- 300g of organic silken tofu

- 1 cup of cashews

- 1 cup of water

- 4 tbsp of cornflour

- 1/2 cup of maple syrup

- 1/4 tsp of Celtic salt

- 1/4 cup of lemon juice

- Medium-ripe pineapple, chopped

Topping:

- 200g of frozen berries

- 1 tbsp of maple syrup

- 1 tbsp of cornflour mixed with 2 tbsp of water

Instructions:

1. For the base, combine desiccated coconut, spelt flour, blended nuts, Celtic salt, maple syrup, and coconut oil. Mix well and press firmly into a dish. Bake at 180°C for about 15 minutes until it turns slightly brown.

2. For the filling, blend silken tofu, cashews, water, cornflour, maple syrup, Celtic salt, and lemon juice in a high-power blender. Pour the mixture into a saucepan and simmer until it thickens. Then pour it over the baked crust to set.

3. For the topping, heat the frozen berries in a saucepan and add cornflour and maple syrup. Stir until it thickens and cook for 2 minutes. Let it cool and then spread it over the set filling. Place the cheesecake in the fridge to chill.

Nutritional Information (per serving, assuming 8 servings): Calories - 439, Protein: 7g, Carbohydrates: 42g, Fat: 29g

Heavenly Fruit-Filled Strudel

Pastry:

- 2 cups of spelt flour (You can use a mix of wholemeal and white)

- 1/2 cup of olive oil

- 1/2 cup of room temperature water

- A pinch of Celtic salt

Pear Cream:

- 1 can (800g) of pears in natural juice or 3 large steamed pears with 1 cup of water

- 3/4 cup of cashews

- 1/4 cup of Brazil nuts

- 1-2 tsp of vanilla extract

- 1 tablespoon of maple syrup (optional)

- A pinch of Celtic salt

Instructions:

1. Form a dough with the pastry ingredients and roll it paper-thin between two sheets of cling wrap.

2. Remove the top piece of cling wrap.

3. Cover the dough with grated apple, a sprinkle of coriander powder, and a drizzle of maple syrup. Add currants and blueberries if desired.

4. Lift one end of the cling wrap and gently fold it. As you continue to lift, the strudel will roll in on itself.

5. Roll the strudel onto a baking dish lined with baking paper.

6. Bake at 200°C for approximately 35 minutes or until it turns golden. Some juices may run out and form a delicious crust. Brush with olive oil or coconut oil if needed before or during cooking. Enjoy this heavenly fruit-filled strudel with pear cream.

Nutritional Information per 1/8th of the strudel: Calories: Approximately 270-350 calories Protein: Approximately 2-4g, Carbohydrates: Approximately 25-40g, Fat: Approximately 18-24g

Plum TeaCake

Ingredients:

280g spelt flour

150g coconut sugar

15g baking powder

Zest from half a lemon

125ml oil

200g soy milk

2 tsp vanilla extract

2 tbsp extra coconut sugar

500g fresh plums (or canned if fresh aren't available)

Instructions:

Grease and line a 10x28cm baking pan and preheat the oven to 160°C (320°F).

Mix all the dry ingredients together, then make a well and add the wet ingredients. You don't need a mixer for this batter. Thinly slice about 200g of fresh plums and gently mix them into the batter.

In the baking tray, evenly sprinkle 2 tablespoons of coconut sugar. Place the halved plums (about 300g) on the bottom of the tray and pour the batter over them.

Bake for an hour, or until a skewer comes out clean. This teacake is light, fluffy, moist, and a healthier dessert option.

Nutritional Information for Plum Teacake: Serving Size - 1 slice. Calories: 200, Fat: 7g, Carbohydrates: 32g, Fiber: 2g, Protein: 3g)

Raw Berry Cheesecake

The Crust:

- 1 cup of raw nuts

- 1 cup of pitted dates

- A pinch of Celtic salt

The Filling:

- 2 cups of raw cashews, soaked overnight, rinsed, and drained

- 1/2 cup of coconut cream

- 1/4 cup of coconut oil

- 1/3 cup of pure maple syrup

- 1/8 cup of lemon juice

- 2 tsp of vanilla extract

- 1/4 tsp of Celtic salt

The Berry Topping (Optional):

- 1 cup of a single type of berry or mixed berries (blueberries, strawberries, raspberries, etc.)

- 2 tbsp of pure maple syrup

Instructions:

1. Prepare the crust by combining the raw nuts, pitted dates, and a pinch of Celtic salt in a food processor. Process until the mixture resembles coarse crumbs and sticks together when pressed.

2. Press the crust mixture firmly into the bottom of a springform pan, creating an even layer. Place the pan in the refrigerator while you work on the filling.

3. To make the filling, blend the soaked and drained raw cashews, coconut cream, coconut oil, pure maple syrup, lemon juice, vanilla extract, and Celtic salt in a high-speed blender. Blend until the mixture is smooth and creamy, scraping down the sides of the blender as needed.

4. Pour the creamy filling over the prepared crust in the springform pan. Smooth the top with a spatula.

5. Place the cheesecake in the freezer to set for at least 4-6 hours, or overnight.

6. Before serving, garnish with fresh berries or make a berry topping by blending your choice of berries with maple syrup until you have a smooth sauce. Drizzle the berry sauce over individual slices of cheesecake.

Nutritional Information (per serving): Calories - 290, Fat: 20g, Carbohydrates: 28g, Fiber: 4g, Protein: 6g

Dairy-Free Cheesecake

Ingredients:

- 680g extra firm tofu

- 1 cup coconut sugar

- 1 tsp vanilla extract

- 1/4 tsp Celtic salt

- 1/4 cup coconut oil

- 2 tbsp lemon juice

- Zest of one lemon

- 2 cups ginger nut biscuit crumbs

Instructions:

1. Preheat your oven to 350°F (160°C) while preparing a 9-inch (23cm) baking tin.

2. Use a tofu press to drain your extra firm tofu, then crumble it into a large mixing bowl.

3. Mix the tofu with coconut sugar, vanilla extract, Celtic salt, coconut oil, lemon juice, and lemon zest.

4. Transfer the mixture into a food processor and blend until smooth.

5. Spread the ginger nut crumbs to form a crust at the bottom of the baking tin.

6. Pour the blended vegan cheesecake mixture onto the crust.

7. Smooth the top layer with a spatula or spoon.

8. Bake in the preheated oven for at least 20 minutes or until the top begins to brown.

9. Once baked, remove the cheesecake and let it cool in the refrigerator.

10. After the cheesecake is chilled, decorate it with assorted berries.

Nutritional Information (per serving): Calories - 320, Fat: 17g, Carbohydrates: 35g, Fiber: 2g, Protein: 6g

Vegan Strawberry Trifle

For the Jelly:

- 10.5 oz strawberries, hulled and cut into small pieces

- 2 tbsp lemon juice

- 4 tbsp maple syrup

- 1 2/3 cups water

- 1 tsp agar agar

- 1 2/3 cups water

For the Custard:

- 3 cups plant-based milk

- 3 tbsp custard powder

- 4 tbsp maple syrup

For the Coconut Whipped Cream:

- 14 oz tin of full-fat coconut milk

- 1 tsp vanilla extract

- 2 tbsp maple syrup

To Decorate (optional):

- Fresh berries

- Pistachio nuts, roughly chopped

Instructions:

For the Jelly:

1. Place the strawberries, lemon juice, maple syrup, and 1 2/3 cups of water in a pan. Cook over low heat for about 10 minutes until the strawberries soften.

2. Use a spoon or fork to gently mash the strawberries against the side of the pan.

3. Add agar agar and mix well, cooking for another couple of minutes until the agar has melted.

4. Pour the jelly mixture into a large trifle dish and allow it to cool and set.

For the Custard:

1. Place the milk in a jar, add the custard powder, and shake well.

2. Pour the milk mixture into a saucepan, add the maple syrup, mix well, and heat on low for a few minutes until thickened. Adjust the thickness with a bit more milk if needed.

3. Pour the custard on top of the set jelly and let it cool to set.

For the Coconut Whipped Cream:

1. Keep a tin of coconut milk in the fridge overnight so the creamy part separates from the watery part at the bottom.

2. Open the tin upside down, pour off the watery liquid, and place the creamy part into a bowl with about 3 tablespoons of the water.

3. Add the maple syrup and vanilla extract.

4. Whip up the coconut cream with an electric whisk until light and fluffy.

To Assemble:

1. Carefully spoon the coconut whipped cream on top of the set custard.

2. Decorate with fresh berries and chopped pistachios if desired.

3. Serve chilled after it has been refrigerated for a few hours.

Nutritional Information (per serving): Calories - 350, Fat: 25g, Carbohydrates: 32g, Fiber: 5g, Protein: 4g

Carob-Infused Black Bean Brownies

Ingredients:

- 850g cooked black beans

- 1/2 cup carob powder

- 1/2 cup spelt flour

- 1/2 cup applesauce

- 1/2 cup maple syrup

- 3 tbsp egg replacer

- 2 tsp vanilla extract

- 1 tsp baking powder

- 1/2 tsp Celtic salt

- 1/2 cup carob chips (optional)

- 1 tsp coffee substitute

Instructions:

1. Preheat the oven to 180°C. Grease and line an 8-inch square baking tin.

2. In a food processor, combine all the ingredients (except carob chips if using) and process until the mixture is completely smooth.

3. Gently fold in the carob chips.

4. Transfer the batter into the prepared cake tin.

5. Bake for 30-35 minutes until the brownies are set but still soft. Let them cool before serving. You can store any leftovers in an airtight container in the fridge for up to 5 days. This recipe makes 9 brownies, making them a great addition to kid's lunch boxes.

Nutritional Information (per serving - 1 brownie): Calories - 300, Fat: 3g, Carbohydrates: 61g, Fiber: 11g, Protein: 12g

Raw Chocolate-Covered Berry Delights

Ingredients:

- 60g cacao butter, finely chopped.

- 1 tablespoon cold-pressed raw organic coconut oil.

- 2 tablespoons raw nut butter or tahini.

- 1 tablespoon pure maple syrup, raw dark agave, or sweetener of your choice.

- 1/4 cup organic raw cacao powder.

- 1/4 tsp vanilla powder (optional).

- Approx. 1 cup frozen organic berries (e.g., raspberries).

Instructions:

1. Melt cacao butter and coconut oil in a glass mixing bowl over boiling water.

2. Remove from heat, add all ingredients except berries, and combine until smooth.

3. Scatter berries into the bottom of small silicone molds or a lined glass dish. Spoon the warm chocolate over the berries, tilting slightly to semi-coat each one. The cold berries will set the chocolate quickly.

4. Refrigerate until needed. These chocolates can be frozen and served from the freezer.

Tips: You can find raw cacao butter, quality raw nut butter, and raw cacao powder at health food stores or online. You can substitute nuts for berries or leave the chocolates plain.

Nutritional Information (per serving - 2 pieces): Calories - 80, Fat: 7g, Carbohydrates: 3g, Fiber: 1g, Protein: 1g

Raw Beetroot Chocolate Cake

Crust:

- 1 cup Brazil nuts

- 1 1/2 cups almonds

- 1 tbsp raw cacao

- 1/4 cup carob powder

- 6 soaked medjool dates (10 minutes in hot water)

Filling:

- 1/2 cup maple syrup

- 1/4 cup raw cacao

- 2 tbsp carob powder

- 3/4 cup coconut oil

- Pinch of Celtic salt

- 2 cups beetroot, peeled and roughly chopped

- 1 1/2 cups pre-soaked raw cashews (about 6 hours)

Topping:

- 1 cup raw cashews

- 1/2 cup coconut oil

- 3 tbsp maple syrup

- 1/4 cup water (or beetroot juice to make it pink or raw cacao for brown)

Instructions:

Crust:

1. Combine all the crust ingredients in a food processor and process until smooth.

2. Sprinkle the carob or cacao powder into the base of a large springform pan and press down the crust mixture. Freeze.

Filling:

1. Blend the maple syrup and beetroot in a blender until very smooth.

2. Add cashews and blend again.

3. Add the remaining ingredients and process. Pour over the frozen base.

4. Cover or seal the cake on a flat surface for about 2 hours in the fridge or freezer until it becomes very firm.

Topping:

1. Process the topping ingredients until very smooth.

2. Pour the mixture over the firm frozen cake, using a flat spatula to spread.

3. Re-freeze for 1-2 hours.

4. Let it sit for 15 minutes before serving. This cake serves 10-12.

Note: Raw cacao is not the same as cocoa. Cacao contains serotonin, tryptophan, tyrosine, and phenylethylamine, which are associated with feelings of wellbeing and happiness.

Nutritional Information (per serving): Calories - 320, Fat: 28g, Carbohydrates: 17g, Fiber: 5g, Protein: 6g

Spiced Apple Pie

Ingredients:

- 2 cups spelt flour

- 1/2 cup olive oil

- 1/2 cup water

- 8 apples (preferably Granny Smith), peeled, cut, cored, and chopped

- 3/4 cup raisins

Instructions:

1. In a mixing bowl, combine the spelt flour, olive oil, and water to form a dough.

2. Use 3/4 of the dough to line a pie pan, reserving the remaining 1/4 for the top crust.

3. Bake the bottom crust in a preheated oven at 350°F (175°C) for about 10 minutes.

4. In a saucepan, stew the chopped apples with just enough water to cover the bottom of the pan. Cook until the apples soften.

5. Add the raisins, cover, and continue stewing until the desired softness is achieved.

6. Transfer the stewed apples and raisins into the pie shell, then cover them with the remaining 1/4 of the pie crust dough.

7. Bake until the pie crust turns golden brown.

8. That's it! While no additional seasonings are used in this recipe, feel free to add your choice of seasonings. Cumin is recommended if you decide to do so.

Nutritional Information (per serving): Calories - 350, Fat: 16g, Carbohydrates: 48g, Fiber: 7g, Protein: 5g

Chocolate and Coconut Chia Pudding

Ingredients:

- 1/2 cup chia seeds

- 1/2 cup dried coconut

- 1/2 cup raw cashews (soaked for 2 hours and drained)

- 2 cups water

- 2 tbsp carob powder

- 1 cup dates

- 1/2 teaspoon vanilla extract

- 1/2 teaspoon lemon juice

- Pinch of salt

Instructions:

1. In a high-speed blender, combine all the ingredients (except for the coconut and chia seeds) and blend until smooth.

2. Pour the mixture into a mixing bowl containing the chia seeds and dried coconut. Stir thoroughly.

3. Let the mixture sit for 5 minutes, then stir it again.

4. Divide the mixture into four dessert bowls and place them in the refrigerator for about half an hour to set.

Nutritional Information (per serving): Calories - 395, Fat: 14g, Carbohydrates: 69g, Protein: 6g

Pomegranate Cheesecake

Ingredients:

Crust:

- 1 cup walnuts

- 1 cup almonds or granola

- 1 cup pitted dates

- Pinch of Celtic salt

Filling:

- 2.5 cups raw cashews (thoroughly washed and soaked for 1 hour)

- 2 1/4 cups pomegranate juice

- 1 tbsp vanilla extract

- 3/4 cup coconut oil

- 1/4 cup lemon juice

- 1/4 tsp salt

- 1/4 cup beet juice or 1/2 small beet

- 1 1/4 cups maple syrup

- 3 tbsp lecithin granules

Instructions:

Crust:

1. Place all crust ingredients in a food processor and mix until the mixture comes away from the edges.

2. Press the mixture firmly into a springform pan to create the crust. Set it aside. (The crust can be made the day before to save time.)

Filling:

1. In a blender, combine all the filling ingredients except for the coconut oil and lecithin. Blend until the mixture is smooth and creamy.

2. Stop blending and add the lecithin and melted coconut oil. Resume blending until the oil and lecithin are well incorporated.

3. Pour the filling into the prepared crust in the springform pan and garnish with pomegranate kernels.

4. Place the cheesecake in the freezer to set for 1-2 hours or overnight.

5. Remove it from the freezer one hour before serving.

6. This recipe makes one 10-inch cheesecake.

Nutritional Information (per serving): Calories - 450, Fat: 29g, Carbohydrates: 42g, Protein: 9g

Baked Apples

Ingredients:

- 4 apples of your choice

- Handful of sultanas

- 2 tbsp coconut sugar

- Handful of pecans

- 4 tbsp coconut oil

- 2 tsp maple syrup

Instructions:

1. Preheat the oven to 380°F (200°C).

2. Carefully score around the circumference of each apple with a small sharp knife.

3. Using an apple corer, remove the core from each apple.

4. In a bowl, mix the sultanas, pecans, and coconut sugar together.

5. Place the apples in a greased and lined baking tin, side by side.

6. Divide the mixture into four portions and press it into the center of each apple.

7. Top each apple with a tablespoon of coconut oil and drizzle with maple syrup.

8. Bake for 20 minutes or until the apples are cooked through. This recipe serves 4.

Nutritional Information (per serving): Calories - 320, Fat: 18g, Carbohydrates: 41g, Protein: 2g

Coconut Pudding with Blueberry Topping

Ingredients for Coconut Pudding:

- 3 cups coconut milk

- 1/2 cup maple syrup

- 1/2 cup cornstarch

- 1/2 cup shredded coconut

- 1/2 teaspoon salt

Instructions for Coconut Pudding:

1. In a saucepan over medium heat, combine all the pudding ingredients.

2. Stir constantly and cook until the mixture thickens.

3. Remove from heat and pour the mixture into a glass pie dish.

4. Cover and refrigerate for a few hours before serving.

Ingredients for Blueberry Topping:

- 4 cups blueberries, fresh or frozen

- 1/2 cup frozen apple juice concentrate

- 1/2 inch of ginger, grated or 1 tsp vanilla extract

Instructions for Blueberry Topping:

1. In a saucepan, combine the blueberries, frozen apple juice concentrate, and grated ginger.

2. Cook for about 10 minutes.

3. Scoop out 1 cup of the mixture and blend it until smooth. Then pour it back into the saucepan and stir well.

4. Chill the topping before serving.

Nutritional Information (per serving): Calories - 275, Fat: 10g, Carbohydrates: 49g, Protein: 2g

Vegan Rice Pudding

Ingredients:

- 1/4 cup maple syrup

- 1 tsp ground coriander

- 5 cups soy milk

- 2 tsp vanilla extract

- 4 cups cooked rice

- 1 cup raw cashews

- 1 tsp Celtic salt

Instructions:

1. Place the cooked rice in a baking dish and set it aside.

2. In a blender, combine the raw cashews, maple syrup, salt, ground coriander, vanilla extract, and 2 cups of soy milk.

3. Blend until you have a smooth mixture.

4. Add the remaining soy milk and blend again.

5. Pour the blended mixture over the rice in the baking dish.

6. Bake for 1 1/2 hours at 180°C/350°F or until the top is brown and puffy.

7. This recipe serves 6.

Nutritional Information (per serving): Calories - 430, Fat: 11g, Carbohydrates: 72g, Protein: 10g

Berry Almond Tea Cake

Ingredients:

- Topping:

- 1/4 cup golden spread

- 2/3 cups spelt flour

- 3 tbsp coconut sugar

- 2 tbsp flaked almonds

- Cake:

  - 2 cups spelt flour

  - 2 tsp baking powder

  - 1/2 tsp bicarbonate soda

  - 1 cup coconut sugar

  - 1 cup almond meal

  - 1/2 cup sunflower oil

  - 1.5 tsp vanilla extract

  - 1/2 tsp almond extract

  - 1 cup soy milk

  - 3/4 cup blackberries

  - 3/4 cup blueberries

Instructions:

1. Preheat your oven to 180°C (350°F) and grease and line a 20cm round cake tin.

2. For the topping, use your fingertips to rub the golden spread into the flour. Stir in the sugar until well combined and set aside.

3. In a large bowl, combine all the dry cake ingredients.

4. In a jug, mix all the wet ingredients and pour them into the dry ingredients.

5. Gently fold the berries into the batter.

6. Pour the batter into the cake tin, smooth the top with a spatula, and add the crumble topping.

7. Cover with foil and bake for 1 hour. Remove the foil and bake for an additional 30 minutes.

8. Once done, remove the cake from the oven and let it cool in the tin. This cake is worth the longer baking time.

9. This recipe serves 10. If you have a thermomix or a good quality food processor, you can powder some coconut sugar and sprinkle it lightly on top.

Nutritional Information (per serving): Calories - 295, Fat: 13g, Carbohydrates: 39g, Protein: 5g

PREPARATIONS

DIY Spice Blend - Curry Powder

Ingredients:
- 2 tablespoons of ground cumin
- 2 tablespoons of ground coriander
- 2 teaspoons of garlic powder
- 2 teaspoons of turmeric
- 2 teaspoons of fenugreek
- 1/2 to 1 teaspoon of cayenne pepper

Instructions:
Mix the ingredients thoroughly. Store the curry powder in a glass jar in your pantry for up to 6 months.

Nutritional Information: This is a seasoning mix, so it doesn't have macronutrients on its own.

Nutty Mince Blend

Ingredients:

- 2/3 cups of sunflower seeds

- 2/3 cups of rolled oats

- 2/3 cups of pecan nuts

- Celtic salt to taste

- 1 teaspoon of dried basil

- 1/4 cup of fresh parsley

Instructions:

1. Start by grinding the sunflower seeds and rolled oats in a food processor until they are well chopped.

2. Dry fry the sunflower seed and rolled oats mixture until it becomes lightly browned.

3. In a separate bowl, mix the ground sunflower seeds and oats with pecan nuts, Celtic salt, dried basil, and fresh parsley.

4. Blend until all the ingredients are well combined.

5. Transfer the Nutty Mince Blend into a ziplock bag and store it in the freezer. This mixture can be stored for up to 3 months and yields approximately 2 1/4 cups.

Nutritional Information (per 1/4 cup): Calories - 180, Protein: 4g, Carbohydrates: 11g, Fat: 15g

Homemade Sourdough Burger Buns

Ingredients:

- 1 cup of active sourdough starter

- 3 tablespoons of coconut oil

- 1/2 cup of water

- 2 tablespoons of honey

- 1 egg

- 1 teaspoon of salt

- 2 - 2 1/2 cups of spelt flour

- 1 egg white

- 1 tablespoon of sesame seeds

Instructions:

1. In a mixing bowl, combine the active sourdough starter, coconut oil, water, honey, and one egg.

2. Gradually add the salt and 2 cups of spelt flour. Continue to add more flour, folding and pressing until you achieve the right consistency. Avoid over-kneading, as spelt flour has lower gluten content. Form the mixture into a ball and cover.

3. Let the dough sit for 1 hour. Stretch, press, or fold it in again and cover.

4. Allow it to sit for 2-6 hours on the counter. For a longer fermentation, you can place it in the fridge overnight, but make sure to bring it to room temperature the following day.

5. Shape the dough into 9 balls, press them to about 1 - 1 1/2 inches thick, and place them on parchment paper. Let them sit for 30 minutes.

6. Mix the egg white and water, brush the buns, and sprinkle them with sesame seeds.

7. Bake for 12-15 minutes at 400 degrees Fahrenheit.

Nutritional Information (per bun, assuming 9 buns): Calories - 226, Protein: 6g, Carbohydrates: 31g, Fat: 9g

Wholesome Gluten-Free Sourdough Loaf

Ingredients:

- 2 teaspoons of salt

- 2 cups of millet flour

- 2 cups of quinoa flour

- 2 cups of buckwheat flour

- 1/4 cup of psyllium husk

- 2 tablespoons of olive oil

- 1-2 cups of buckwheat starter (bring it to room temperature if stored in the fridge)

Instructions:

1. In a large bowl, combine salt, water, and the buckwheat starter. Mix well to dissolve the salt.

2. Add millet flour, quinoa flour, and olive oil. Stir until well mixed.

3. Add psyllium husk to the mixture and continue mixing until the dough has a thick cake batter-like consistency. You may need to adjust the consistency with a little more water or flour.

4. Transfer the dough into a well-oiled bread tin. Optionally, sprinkle some sesame seeds inside the bread tin and on top of the dough after lightly oiling it. Cover with a lid or cling wrap.

5. Allow the dough to rise for 3-4 hours until it increases in height by about one-third to half its original size. Avoid over-rising as it may collapse in the oven.

6. Bake in a preheated oven at 180°C (350°F) for 1.5 hours. You can cover the bread tin with foil during the first hour to prevent over-drying or excessive browning.

7. Once baked, remove the loaf from the tin and let it cool on a rack. For easier slicing, wait until the bread is cold. Enjoy your gluten-free sourdough bread.

Nutritional Information (per serving, assuming 12 servings): Calories - 206, Protein: 4g, Carbohydrates: 35g, Fat: 6g

Easy Sourdough Starter for Beginners

(Yield: Approximately 240g)

- 3/4 Glass jar

- Spelt flour

- Warm water

Instructions:

This starter will take around 7 days in warm temperatures, and up to 2 weeks for a strong starter.

DAY 1: In a large jar, combine 1/2 cup of spelt flour and 1/4 cup of warm water (about 85F). Mix thoroughly with a fork until smooth, creating a thick, pasty mixture. Cover with cling wrap or a lid and let it rest in a warm spot at around 75F for 24 hours.

DAY 2: Check for any bubbles on the surface and let it rest for another 24 hours. If you see a dark liquid called "hooch," don't worry; leave it for now, and you can remove it the next day.

DAY 3: Remove and discard half of your starter, leaving about 60g (1/2 cup). The texture will be stretchy. Add 1/2 cup of flour and 1/4 cup of warm water to the jar. Mix until it resembles thick pancake batter. Cover and rest in a warm spot for another 24 hours.

DAYS 4, 5 & 6: Continue feeding your starter by removing and discarding half of it and adding 1/2 cup of flour and 1/4 cup of warm water each day. As the yeast develops, your starter will rise, form bubbles, and get fluffy. When it falls, it's time to feed it again.

DAY 7: Your starter should have doubled in size with large and small bubbles. It should have a pleasant smell and not be stinky. If these conditions are met, your starter is ready to use.

LAST STEP: Transfer the starter to a clean jar. If you bake often, store your starter at room temperature and feed it 1-2 times a day. If you bake occasionally, store it in the fridge and feed it once a week. When storing in the fridge, there's no need to bring it to room temperature before feeding; just give it flour and water and return it to the fridge.

Simple Spelt Sourdough Bread

(Recipe in grams for accuracy)

Ingredients:

- 65g active sourdough starter

- 315g warm water (80F)

- 10g runny honey or maple syrup

- 240g white spelt flour

- 200g wholemeal spelt flour

- 9g Celtic salt

Instructions:

1. In a large bowl, whisk together the active sourdough starter, warm water, and honey. Add the flours, starting with a fork or spatula and then switching to your hands. Mix until you have a rough, sticky dough without any dry bits. Sprinkle the salt on top, cover with a damp towel, and let it rest for 1 hour (this is the autolyse).

2. After the autolyse, work the dough with your hands, squeezing and kneading for at least 2 minutes to start building gluten. Perform your first set of stretch and folds and let the dough rest for 30 minutes, covered.

3. Perform additional sets of stretch and folds, resting for 30 minutes between each set.

4. Cover the dough with a damp towel and let it rise until it's about 75% increased in size, with small bubbles throughout and a slight jiggle in the bowl. This depends on how the dough looks rather than time.

5. Shape the dough as desired and let it go through its final rise on the countertop until it's almost doubled.

6. Preheat your oven to 475F. Cover the dough with parchment paper, place a cutting board on top, and flip onto the counter so the seam is on the parchment. Gently rub some flour on top and score the dough.

7. Place the dough in a dutch oven and bake at 450F for 25 minutes with the lid on. Remove the lid, reduce the heat to 435F, and bake for an additional 20 minutes or until the exterior is golden brown and crispy.

8. Allow the bread to cool for an hour before cutting. Store it in a plastic bag, cut side down for up to four days.

Homemade Almond Milk

Ingredients:

- 1 cup raw almonds (soaked overnight in cool water, or 1-2 hours in very hot water)

- 5 cups filtered water (use less for thicker milk or more for a thinner consistency)

- 1 pinch of Celtic salt

- 2 whole dates (optional for sweetness)

- 1 tsp vanilla extract (optional for flavor)

Instructions:

1. Add all ingredients to a high-speed blender and blend until the mixture is creamy and smooth. It's best to run the blender for at least 1-2 minutes to fully extract the almond goodness.

2. Strain the mixture using a nut milk bag, squeezing it to extract all the liquid. You can save the leftover almond pulp for baking, especially in crackers.

3. Transfer the almond milk to a jar or bottle and refrigerate. It will stay fresh for 4-5 days but is best when consumed fresh. Be sure to shake it well before drinking, as it can separate. This recipe yields approximately 5 cups.

Nutritional Information (per serving): Calories - 30, Fat: 3g, Carbohydrates: 1g, Protein: 1g

Homemade Coconut Milk & Cream

Ingredients:

- For Light Coconut Milk:

  - 4 cups water

  - 1 cup shredded dried coconut

- For Regular Coconut Milk:

  - 4 cups water

  - 2 cups shredded dried coconut

- For Thick Coconut Milk:

  - 4 cups water

  - 3 cups shredded dried coconut

- For Coconut Cream:

  - 4 cups water

  - 4 cups shredded dried coconut

Instructions:

1. Place the respective quantity of shredded dried coconut and water in a high-powered blender.

2. Blend for 1-2 minutes until the coconut is thoroughly pulverized. You may need to blend for 3-5 minutes with certain blenders.

3. Do not sweeten or add flavorings until you've strained the milk from the pulp.

4. Strain the mixture through a nut bag or muslin cloth, squeezing out as much milk as possible.

5. You can use the leftover pulp in other recipes like smoothies, crusts, cookies, crackers, cakes, or raw bread.

6. Flavor your milk after removing the pulp. Add sweeteners, vanilla or any flavor extract, or carob powder if desired.

7. Store the milk in an airtight glass container for 3-5 days in the fridge. You can also freeze it in ice cube trays for adding to smoothies.

Nutritional Information (per serving of regular coconut milk): Calories - 120, Fat: 12g, Carbohydrates: 4g, Fiber: 2g, Protein: 2g

Homemade Soy Milk

Ingredients:

- 1/2 cup dried soybeans

- 4 cups water

- 1/2 tsp vanilla extract

- 4 dates (optional)

Instructions:

1. Soak the soybeans in water overnight, ideally for 12 hours or longer. Drain the soybeans and remove the outer skins for better texture (optional).

2. Blend the soaked and peeled soybeans with 3 cups of water until well blended and almost smooth.

3. Strain the mixture using a nut milk bag, cheesecloth, napkin, or a fine mesh strainer.

4. Pour the mixture into a pot, add 1 cup of water, and bring it to a boil, stirring occasionally. Skim off any foam.

5. Cook over medium heat for about 20 minutes.

6. Allow the soy milk to cool. You can add vanilla extract or dates for flavor.

7. Store any leftovers in a sealed container in the fridge.

Nutritional Information (per serving): Calories - 70, Fat: 2g, Carbohydrates: 7g, Protein: 5g

Cashew Parmesan

Ingredients:

- 1/2 cup raw cashews

- 1/2 tsp garlic powder

- 1/2 tsp stock powder

- 1/2 tsp Celtic salt

Instructions:

1. Combine all the ingredients and pulse until they resemble the texture of Parmesan cheese.

2. Store the cashew Parmesan in an airtight container in the refrigerator for up to 6 weeks.

3. This recipe yields 2/3 cup, and a serving size is approximately 1 teaspoon.

Nutritional Information (per serving): Calories - 9, Fat: 1g, Carbohydrates: 1g, Protein: 0g

NOTES

About PrimeInsight Press

At PrimeInsight Press, our story begins as a passionate small team with a belief: knowledge, when shared with passion, can change the world. We have dedicated ourselves to creating enlightening workbooks, authentic, and professional guides, also paying special attention to their high-quality, engaging interior design.

We believe that every workbook is an opportunity to touch hearts and empower minds. Through the pages of our workbooks, we hope to inspire you to dream and provide you with the tools to bring those dreams to life.

Join us at PrimeInsight Press, and together, transform your journey of growth, one page at a time.

Thank you for purchasing this book.

If you enjoyed it, please leave a brief review. Your feedback is important to us and will help other readers decide whether to read the book too.

For a small company like us, getting reviews (especially on Amazon) means a lot to us.

We can't THANK YOU enough for this!

Important Notice

We take customer suggestions seriously. If you have any, please write to:primeinsightpress@gmail.com and include the book's title in the email subject.

Made in the USA
Las Vegas, NV
03 December 2023

82046854R00077